I0093115

Confronting Dementia

*A Husband's Journey as
an Alzheimer's Caregiver*

Stu Ervay

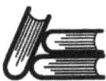

EABooks Publishing
Your Partner In Publishing

Copyright @ 2021 Stu Ervay

All rights reserved. No part of this publication may be reproduced or transmitted in any form or by any electronic or mechanical means including photo copying, recording, or any information storage and retrieval system now known or to be invented, without permission in writing from the publisher or the author.

Scripture quotations marked (KJV), are from The Holy Bible, King James Version. The KJV is in public domain.

Name: Stu Ervay
Title: Confronting Dementia: A Husband's Journey as an Alzheimer's Caregiver
LCCN: 2021908794
ISBN: 978-1-952369-72-8
Subjects: 1. FAMILY & RELATIONSHIPS/ Lifestages/Later Years
2. HEALTH & FITNESS / DISEASE/Alzheimers & Dementia
3. SELF HELP / Death/Grief/Bereavement

Interior Design by Darryl Bennett
Cover Design by Robin Black
Front Cover Photo Credit: iStockphoto/monkeybusinessimages
Back Cover Photo Credit: iStockphoto/a_Taiga

Published by EA Books Publishing, a division of
Living Parables of Central Florida, Inc. a 501c3

EABooksPublishing.com

Table of Contents

REFLECTIONS AS A CAREGIVING HUSBAND

CAREGIVING CHALLENGES OTHERS FACE

*COMMENTARIES ON LIVING DURING
A CAREGIVING CHALLENGE*

Foreword

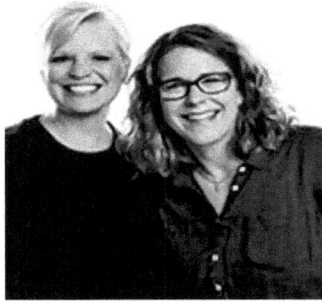

We had the pleasure of meeting Dr. Ervay and his wife, Barbara, about four years ago as he contemplated placing her in one of our care homes. Through our work with people living with dementia we have found a profound difference in the impact of caring for a spouse, rather than a parent who is living with dementia. The process they go through in turning over the care of their wife or husband can be grueling. Riddled with guilt, and self-doubt.

In his book, Dr. Ervay captures the essence of the bond of marriage and the devastating toll that a diagnosis of Alzheimer's or another dementia can take. Although there is no definitive cause or cure, there is much written about the deterioration process happening within. Scans of healthy brains compared with "Alzheimer's Brains" show without a doubt the ravage of this disease on the body. A lesser explored topic is the toll that this process takes on the surviving spouse.

As the owners of Prairie Elder Care, we strive to provide nurturing support for the spouse, understanding that the plagues of the elderly: loneliness, helplessness and boredom are likely impacting them as well. Although the pandemic has greatly impeded our ability to provide this support in person, supporting the caregiver has been a foundational element of our work.

Prairie Elder Care consists of four group homes with eight residents living in each. Our mission is giving back community, connection and control to our residents and their loved ones. Our desire is to provide top-notch physical care, and to care for the emotional and spiritual needs of our residents and their families. We invest a great deal in ensuring that we have enough caregiving and nursing staff to keep a close eye on the well-being of each of our residents. Nurses communicate regularly with families and know the residents well enough to discern even the smallest of changes in their conditions. This robust model keeps families feeling in control and allows them to spend their time enjoying their loved one rather than putting out fires.

When we met Dr. Ervay, and he learned more about our approach, we will never forget his comment that our is work every bit a ministry as much as a business. Our hope is to leave a legacy that changes the landscape of dementia care and support for families. In our book and engagement model, *Now is Found*, we discuss education as a means for impacting the stigma of dementia and improving the care of those living with it.

As both Stu and Barbara are educators, we are, too, working to shed light on the impact of this disease and improve the lives of those in its path. We have extended our work in residential care, to providing day program services for people who are still at home. For spouses who are still able to have their loved one at home, a time of respite each week can be priceless. We understand that this disease leaves a trail of heartbreak and destruction. The loss is not only experienced by the person living with the disease, but maybe even more so by spouses and other family members.

As Dr. Ervay puts it, the loved one is becoming a "human being with no dynamic inner core." This process may be more difficult to watch than to directly experience.

Our goal is to be a non-judgmental guide through the healthcare side of the process as well as someone who can share in the grief, loss, and heartache. We also take our role as stewards of joy and positivity very seriously! As a part of our mission, we hold classes for family caregivers to educate them about the progression of the disease, as well as provide strategies for staying connected.

While we pursue our mission of giving back community, connection and control, one of the common outcomes is the ability for family members to find better ways to connect with their loved one. With a focus on creating a feeling of control for the person living with dementia, they are better able to make connections with the people and environment around them. As stronger connections are made between residents, staff caregivers and families, we develop a feeling of community that not only benefits our residents, but their loved ones too.

Exactly one month before we were forced to close our doors to visitors due to COVID-19, we held a Valentine's dinner for all the couples involved in Prairie Elder Care. We transported our residents to our community center, and their spouses met them there. They were waited on by our staff, served a delicious candlelight meal, and celebrated. For some it was the last meal they would eat together.

The pandemic has highlighted the need to go beyond just the physical care, but also tend to the emotional and spiritual needs of our elders. Now is the time to consider the shortcomings of our traditional model and explore how to care for this population so they can thrive and experience a dignity that is more that just a physical existence.

Through his beloved wife, Barbara, Stu continues their legacy of educating and making the world better for others. This book has the potential to impact not only married couples, but to also bring a new level of understanding to extended families. His intimate sharing of his experience opens the door to shine a light on the challenges faced by a surviving spouse, and the importance of including family caregivers in the process.

In the end, we share the hope that these stories contribute to a new focus on improving the lives of so many impacted by this disease.

Mandy Shoemaker, MEd
Michala Gibson, BSN

Introduction

Alois Alzheimer, a German psychiatrist and neuropathologist, lived between 1864 and 1915. He was the scientist who gave his name to a rare condition discovered at the turn of the twentieth century. His research findings made a distinction between senile dementia and a new form of cognitive dysfunction that appeared in younger people.

By the middle of the twentieth century the condition with Alzheimer's name had grown exponentially. Not just early onset but in people much older. Today it is a worldwide epidemic. Its causes are unknown and unfortunately, there is no cure.

My wife, who suffered from mild epilepsy from age fourteen, began having symptoms associated with dementia soon after turning seventy. By age seventy-six her symptoms were challenging our family and me. A year later we were forced to admit her to a residential care facility.

The diagnosis: Alzheimer's.

Our fiftieth wedding anniversary occurred in 2012. The family made it special. With help, my wife and I were able to take some memory-lane trips up to five years after the celebration. And for the most part, we continued a normal life.

My life as an Alzheimer's caregiver is not unique. Nor has it been overly stressful when compared to similar stories. Interactions with other caregivers and my volunteer work with AARP have given me additional insights. As a planner for the future, I work at staying healthy, fit and mentally focused.

I have made mistakes and still do. This caregiving situation depresses me, with occasional bouts of despair. But they are just exaggerated sensations of what we all experience in ordinary life. Peaks and valleys in our emotional affiliation with living. I have been lucky. Some would prefer "blessed."

Writing is one of my hobbies. Which is why I offer my insights:

- To help other husbands in a similar situation.
- To be a tribute to my wife and our decades of life together.
- To help me climb out of the emotional valleys I occasionally fall into.

Confronting Dementia

Dementia is a generic word that covers many cognitive dysfunctions. Alzheimer's Disease is just one of them. Others include Dementia with Lewy Bodies, Vascular Dementia, Frontotemporal Dementia, Parkinson's Disease Dementia, Pick's Disease, and Creutzfeldt-Jakob Disease. Individuals may suffer from more than one type, referred to as Mixed Dementia.

The symptoms for each kind of dementia vary. Partially due to the characteristics of the disorder. Or because of the individual's baseline personality. Behaviors change as disorders progress: depression, forgetfulness, confusion, anger, suicidal tendencies, intense stubbornness, docility, and others.

Afflicted individuals become increasingly unable to negotiate their way through the disorder. Unlike people suffering from diseases and disorders which do not directly affect the brain. Those individuals can assist in caring for themselves and communicate with helpers.

All caregiving is challenging. But it is especially difficult when the afflicted person, once alive and even vivacious, seems to mentally disappear.

Little by little. Becoming a human being with no dynamic inner core.

That phenomenon is especially difficult for a husband who genuinely loves his wife. As he once knew her. A complete person, helpmate, confidant, compassionate supporter, an intelligent and witty companion. An emotional shelter when the world "outside" seemed to be collapsing around us. Many men do not want to admit how deeply affected they are by what is happening to their wives. I am no exception.

Some think it is like losing an arm or a leg. Then figuring out how to manage without that limb.

But it is not at all like that. It is more like losing a part of your body that makes you who you are. And the pain never goes away. No crutches or prosthetics will replace the missing part.

A little piece of your life has been extracted, will never regrow, and cannot be replaced.

Nevertheless, coping is necessary. How a husband copes depends on many factors:

- His basic personality.
- Characteristics of the relationship he had with his wife in normal times.
- Enculturation both before and during the marriage.
- The strength of his biological family and interactions with friends.
- The closeness he continues to share with associates and the community of which he is a part.

The physical and mental health of the husband is another strong consideration. And the extent to which that health is supported by personal habits, moral and religious beliefs, and activities that give hope to his future.

A reason for living, as his wife fades away.

Diversions or hobbies certainly help. But they offer only a temporary respite unless they are part of a larger pattern of involvement. Something of a continuum in which others are involved.

Confronting dementia is difficult for anyone. Children, siblings, other relatives, and close friends. But the confrontation is more significant and difficult with spouses. Married people in healthy relationships are bonded in special intimate ways.

The obvious is physical, but in time that connection becomes less important. Bonding is a mysterious thing that incorporates soulful understandings, a merging of spiritual and emotive interrelations. When the bond is broken or weakened, the spouse left behind becomes different. It is that condition this book addresses.

Evolution of the Book

This book began as a blog titled *Alzheimer's and the Husband*. Although I have written extensively in my career as educator and university professor, blogging involves a unique writing style. I found a wonderful editor who has guided me through the process.

Blogging is not a structured activity in which there is a continuous story line. Those who write blogs follow a theme. But individual submissions (posts) are not necessarily chapters. Rather, they are expansions and elaborations on the theme.

Transforming my blog into this book required me to reorganize and reformat. As I wrote, I had continuity in mind. The elements of that continuity followed a logical thread that started with *my own reflections as a caregiving husband*. After pursuing that direction, I examined and commented on *caregiving challenges others faced*.

Then I created stories about them. Stories different than mine. Situations I knew by spending time with other caregivers. Or reading about their challenges. Scenarios were first introduced that presented unique situations. Then I created fictitious couples who became characters in those stories.

The stories did not have happy endings. There is nothing happy about a diagnosis of Alzheimer's. But, after telling the stories, I reflected on how outcomes might have been better. *The last posts in the blog were commentaries on how we can manage living during a caregiving challenge.*

The book is formatted essentially the same way, using three separate categories:

- My experiences
- The experiences of others
- Commentaries on caregiving

To keep the cohesiveness of the book's contents, I focused on something specific. Usually a word or phrase that had the potential to be meaningful. Even powerful. With each blog post, I selected a word that applied to a theme I wished to pursue in the context of my own understandings, the experiences of others, and the effect caregiving has on those who provide it.

Below are the words I used and why I used them for each post. Now they have become chapters in this book, summarized under each of the three categories I created.

My Experiences

ALWAYS: Young and healthy adults think of life as blissful eternity. Coming to the realization of "always" as a temporary kind of euphoria is difficult to acknowledge. But acknowledge it we must.

PASSION: Worthwhile lives are built on passion. A uniquely human emotion that overrides basic needs, providing purpose and meaning for our time on earth. Passion multiplied by two, a man and a woman with compatible enthusiasms, is fulfillment writ large.

LEGACY: Time and space, no matter how they are defined by science, seem infinite to us. We are not infinite in terms of our senescent existence on earth. But all of us leave a legacy to our fellow human beings. Big or small. Good or bad. Short or lasting. Legacies can manifest as things, ideas, improvements, insights, and revelations. The most significant legacy may be love.

LONELINESS: Loneliness is an American epidemic, made worse by the COVID–19 pandemic and social unrest. It can be defined as a disorientation. Not knowing how or why to live when a spouse fades away in the fog of Alzheimer's or any other debilitating disorder. When familial, intimate, or even social contact is nearly extinct. When life's meaning becomes obscure or confusing.

ALONENESS: It is difficult to do or believe the right thing when others find your behavior unacceptable according to their standards. It is even more difficult when you are different from others. When you are shunned or otherwise dismissed. Moral, reasonable, and sensitive convictions, when applied to the service of others, transcends contravening beliefs. A worthy legacy even for the one left after Alzheimer's diminishes the supportive power of two minds and hearts working in concert.

ENGAGEMENT: The definition of engagement can be split into two parts: *ordinary* and *intense*. I focus on "intense." Ordinary engagements such as those associated with hobbies, games, sports, relaxation, conversation, sightseeing travel, parties, entertainment, and dinner are not wrong. Intense engagement is related to serious involvement, whether physical, emotional, or intellectual. All three types can be described in various ways. The one I find most satisfying is intellectual, so I write intensely. Reading, studying, and reflecting can also be intense. These behaviors do not dominate my life's balance, nor did they dominate my marriage. But engagement in the context of ideas and deep understanding is an important core of who we are as human beings. What my wife and I were as a couple. What that legacy gives to me today.

FAITH: Expressions of faith vary. Even within the Christian community. The role faith plays in supporting my caregiving is not easy to explain. For some people faith in God is scripturally clear and absolute. Prayer and devotion are straightforward. Like some others, my religious beliefs are comforting but complicated. From an ecclesiastical point-of-view, my approach to faith is through apologetics. By building a case for my beliefs, as C. S. Lewis did, I eventually reach a point in which my grieving is mitigated through a spiritual connection.

GENDER: We are all human beings that function the same way when it comes to caregiving. But with a few variations. In our culture, distinctions are often gender related. The assumption is that women, being more maternal, are better caregivers. There is some truth in that belief. However, the crossover point may be in preparing and implementing a plan. My wife and I discussed those topics years ago. Managing finances, building support networks, and answering all the "what ifs" as we realistically considered the future. Caregiving fails when people purposely or inadvertently ignore the realities of life.

RELATIONSHIPS: Men need quality relationships as much as women. We need relationships that cover the spectrum of our emotions, that range from buddy-talk to an exploration of how we feel about our worthiness, spiritual beliefs, the purpose of our lives, and sense of acceptance by others. Many stories about caregiving men include addictions to alcohol or drugs, shutdowns emotionally and physically, or going mentally haywire. Somehow, they convince themselves there is no other escape from the horrific psychological battles that challenge them. A kind of caregiving PTSD. And their own aging makes the problem worse, as they acknowledge the loss of ego and sense of being valued by others. They need quality relationships, not the superficial and commercial kinds of assistance touted in today's marketplace.

The Experiences of Others

This series of chapters introduces the importance of acknowledging differences in caregiving stories. Just as the effects of Alzheimer's can vary depending on the individual's personality and life experiences, so too can the thread of day-to-day life of a caregiving man or couple. Much depends on what each brought into the marriage, the lifelong dynamics of that relationship, cultural biases and perspectives, the extent to which they shared a mutually felt purpose, and effective planning for the end-of-life scenario.

These snippets include titles meant to provoke a recognition of where the story starts and might end. Through these descriptors it is possible to see why unique problems may surface once a wife contracts Alzheimer's:

- Real Men are Not Whiners
- Success in Life is Multifaceted
- God is Ever Present in Our Lives
- Marriage is a Necessary Burden
- Institutionalization is Unacceptable
- Too Young, Too Soon, Too Burdensome
- PTSD Multiplied
- Follow the Money

Subsequent chapters speaking to those topics are given names of fictitious men and couples with stories that relate to one or more of the above scenarios. Interspersed among those stories are discussions of the circumstances involved and how those endings might have been different.

Commentaries on Caregiving

The final chapters are summarizing viewpoints.

CONTINGENCIES: This chapter details mindsets such as how we can work to avoid becoming victims. How we can, in some ways, control our own destinies. It is possible to avoid shrugging our shoulders and let fate take its course. We begin with understanding how the world, and the human beings in it, realistically operate. Not just being a Pollyanna. But negotiating our way through challenges the best we can, while acknowledging the possibility we might not be able to pull it off. By devising and using strategies to meet obstacles, we have a better chance of managing crises like Alzheimer's.

HAPPINESS: The word happiness seems meaningful to us, but we often do not know what it really is. In our own lives. On our own terms. Within the guidelines set for us by the society in which we live. Americans cherish *freedom*. Freedom is supposed to make us happy. But freedom as an action is loaded with unknowns, so the only way to work through those unknowns is to create a personal pathway. Happiness requires a certain amount of self-discipline and acknowledgement that our lives are intertwined with all other people. Including those we care for who have Alzheimer's.

WE: Human beings are social animals. We need each other and want to be together. Pandemics and other forces that curtail this opportunity range from inconveniences to emotional traumas. One-to-one connection is almost imperative for us, which makes virtual contact a distant "second best." But simply being together is not enough. We must share a common cause. We must be part of something larger than ourselves. Working to ensure a common cause is worthwhile and uplifting. So, I choose to serve a larger mission in addition to taking care of myself and managing the care of a wife with Alzheimer's.

MENTORING: We need role models. People we can emulate. People who teach us how to live responsibly and happily. And how to be of service to others. Mentoring does not come from just one or two persons. It comes from all those we admire—those who are resourceful and even self-sufficient. But self-sufficiency should not include becoming totally untethered from the support of others. It is essentially the avoidance of victimhood. To seek and accept the assistance of others but never accede willy-nilly to their advice. The practice of good mentoring seeks the development of a stronger self in others. Especially in the caregiving world. Particularly with Alzheimer's.

BELONGING: The sense of belonging involves much more than human beings clustered together. It is a mix of purposeful enterprise, overcoming challenges, making the impossible possible, failing and overcoming that failure, and participating in the building of something remarkable. Perhaps this is the reason why so many of the so-called "Greatest Generation" think back on World War II with nostalgia. The war was a blemish on humanity, but it changed America by enhancing our sense of belonging to something meaningful. Caregivers need that sense of belonging, because they are part of a network of people facing awful challenges. And they prevail because of that supportive network.

RESOURCEFULNESS: Resourcefulness has a range of meanings. For me it is related mostly to common sense, but dictionaries use synonyms such as ingenious, gifted, and vigorous. All those definitions include the ability to stay on top of things. "Not letting the gremlins grind you down," to paraphrase a colleague. Avoiding emotional paralysis. Finding the wherewithal to tackle problems one step at a time, yet never losing sight of the ultimate objective. If we chip away at problems a little at a time, then time itself can be part of the solution. Caring for a beloved wife with Alzheimer's must be one of life's most difficult challenges, but it is another marital obligation AND a loving opportunity. We just need to allow our resourcefulness to emerge and solve the problems day by day, moment by moment.

PURPOSE: Woven through this book are references to purpose. Why have we been given life and what are we supposed to do with it? Thousands of books and other media have been created in the attempt to answer this question, most of which are related to religion. But we gain personal insight into the meaning of the word through many influences. Four of them are mentioned: family, culture, aptitude, and values. Purpose is not simply an attachment to our personalities. It becomes inherent to who we are, what we think, and how we act. And, at least theoretically, we live in a society that gives us the freedom to fulfill our purpose as we see fit. This chapter introduces the idea of "tweaking" an ingrained purpose or modifying it to meet the challenge of caring for a wife with Alzheimer's.

CULTURE: Although context can be multifaceted, culture must be defined within context. Family, our social environment, time and place. All those influences make us who and what we are. It is possible to learn in ways that modify those influences. I have learned to be somewhat different than the culture into which I was born, but with much overlap. Sometimes the overlapping elements conflict, yet most of the time they are mutually supportive. To be aware of our cultural characteristics is important in any context. But critical in the caring of a wife with Alzheimer's.

APTITUDE: Some educators and parents think aptitude has only one dimension. That it has everything to do with a young person's ability to succeed in school. In this chapter the word aptitude is given a much deeper meaning. Educators are beginning to realize aptitude is an internal shapeshifter, never just one thing for all time. A person's *aptitude below the surface* is not identified by the number indicated on a test. Such an aptitude is often a willingness to accept responsibility at levels no pencil and paper test can ever discern. It is the dynamic quality that lies under the visible personality. Aptitude supports the acceptance of responsibility needed to become a caregiver for someone else. Such as a wife with Alzheimer's.

VALUES: Competition and winning are American values. And those values are consistently tested. Success in the competitive arena can result in the acquisition of wealth, power, and influence. An age-old story from many societies and civilizations. If we are not winners, we are losers. The value of winning becomes an across-the-board principle. In war, sports, board games, even social status. But in this chapter winning is defined as a valued principle when it *means something*—when human existence is elevated and revered. When lives are saved and uplifted until the inevitable laws of nature win. Alzheimer's always wins no matter what we do. But WE win when we hold on and support each other through love, empathy, and service.

The end of the book includes suggestions. Some readers may want to read those first. As in, *let's skip the buildup and get to the point*. But sometimes the buildup *is* the point. Or the reflective foundation that supports it.

When I was young it seemed that reflection was a waste of time. Do it this way or that way. But when it comes to taking care of a wife with Alzheimer's, that philosophy is full of holes. Reflection is not just an action or set of actions. Rather, it involves a full-blown set of demeanors and an emergence of the inner core of who we are as men.

That is the point of this book. Men do not like to admit to having vulnerabilities. But we do. Lots of them. So, it is how we overcome those perceived deficiencies that make us the kinds of husbands we want to be. To be there for the women we love most. To take care of that wife as completely as possible in her time of great need. When she suffers from Alzheimer's.

And thus, to survive the ordeal ourselves.

Chapter 1
Always

A young woman and man begin their magical journey together as a couple. They date, court, commit, and vow to love and care for each other always.

"Always" has a nice ring to it. Kind of like *eternally*. Similar to a fairytale in which Prince Charming and Cinderella live happily ever after. Neither of them will die.

If one gets sick or injured, the other will mend the wounds and whisper words of comfort, expressions of eternal devotion, and declarations of unswerving fidelity.

We all need beautiful aspirations. Relationships, no matter how they begin, are founded on hope and a faith that somehow the fairytale will come true. It is possible none of us would enter any relationship if hope did not exist.

We must have faith that something in our world, such as its maker or guardian, will watch over us and help us be exceptional. Faith in the good thing that comes next is the root of our happiness.

As time passes in our relationship, we realize exceptionality or even survival requires more than the loving touch of a power beyond our knowing. Relationships are what we work to make them.

Unfortunately, there is nothing physically eternal about them. All living things, and the conditions in which they exist, will ultimately fade away and disappear. That is the deal.

C.S. Lewis and his wife worked their way together through her cancer and eventual death. To capture and hold on to every minute. To accept the fact that living our lives to the fullest is not for the faint of heart.

We simply do the best we can for as long as we can. And we are grateful.

I've noticed that personally sensitive topics are rarely covered in books by men. Especially men my age. But at age eighty-two and in a marriage of nearly fifty-eight years, I have learned a few things about faith, love, loss, caregiving and the real meaning of loyalty and devotion.

What I have learned includes, but also transcends religious beliefs, social mores, community expectations, and the real meaning of commitment. I have also come to understand my own gender-related behaviors as they pertain to grieving, seeking solace, and searching for the support and understanding of others.

Why have those revelations hit me now? Because Alzheimer's gives new meaning to the word *always*. It hatches and festers out of sight, then continuously emerges from the inner workings of what was once a vital and active mind. It resolutely seeps into a personality, coming to the surface unexpectedly, taking on bizarre shapes and behaviors.

At first, I did not recognize it for what it was. But I learned it was an ongoing presence that refused to go away. Alzheimer's convinces everyone who loves the afflicted person that it is perpetual and pervasive, until death stops its steady march.

The years slip by. Years once set aside for travel and discovery. Instead they are increasingly filled with opportunities for the "one" to be a loving and competent caregiver, doing all that can be done to spark an old memory or new awareness. A routine is maintained, yet surprises are expected and planned for.

Often, my wife was puzzled by my behavior. Her disease required me to put safety locks on doors, hire people to stay in the house when I ran errands, and incompetently prepare meals when everyone knew I was a lousy cook.

Alzheimer's insisted that I, the other one, make decisions I did not want to make. Decisions made independently in a home in which decisions had always been arrived at together.

Alzheimer's builds walls that seem to have a life of their own. Sometimes they seem to shrink, only to grow an hour later. Rationality becomes a kind of oxymoron, like saying that people afflicted with dementia think logically. Sometimes they do and sometimes they do not. The one who lives in the past, who was the other half of "we" can become confused, sometimes even angry.

It does not help when an outside observer, compassionately motivated or not, says "She can't help it." Of course, she can't. But where did that woman I married go? Where is the woman who stood up and said "always" like I did? Is "always" a lie?

Vowing to remain forever as one body was plausible during eras in which earthly life spans were comparatively short. The afterlife was accepted as everlasting. It made sense when people depended on marriage as an inviolable foundation for survival in harsh cultures and challenging times. Death was just around the corner. When it came, it was usually swift and a gateway to heavenly bliss.

Welcome to the twenty-first century, an era in which nothing is fixed in the realm of faith, the nature of unconditional love, or in distinguishing between fairytales and real life. Technology, medical science, advances in biology, and the growth of social media give "always" a new look.

And sometimes that "look" is harsh and unsettling.

Chapter 2
Passion

My father was my role model: a good provider, handyman, mechanic, and creative inventor. He often reflected on what could be. His idea of raising sons was to keep us involved in interesting, even challenging projects. Dad often started building something in our little shop then let us continue working on it using our own ideas after he went to work.

He taught us how to think. In many ways he was a downhome example of what George Bernard Shaw said: You see things; and you say, "Why?" But I dream things that never were; and I say, "Why not?"[1]

Dad believed society and how we relate to one another could stand improvement. Beyond mere interest or enthusiasm. It was his total passion. And I became imbued with a similar passion.

Dad was not talented in explaining the birds and bees. We had no sister. Girls were kind of alien versions of ourselves who lived in another social universe. In the 1950s our passions and girls' passions were like ships passing in the night.

Dad said our attitudes would change when we grew into our later teens. He was right, of course. In my junior and senior years of high school I experienced an attitude adjustment when it came to girls. A biologically inevitable condition.

One day during my teens Dad waxed philosophical about my future. He assumed I would soon look around for a wife. No. At that time girls were just pleasant diversions for me with no crossover of fundamental interests.

"That will change," Dad said, "especially as you mature and start dating women of substance and conviction. The glue that binds a man and woman together is as much an outwardly directed passion as the physical and emotional passion we feel for each other."

Upon graduation from college, I was commissioned as an army officer. While in the army I met a woman of substance and conviction. We talked and talked about what we could contribute to make our world a better place. The crossover was our common interest in education. Education became our platform for service.

I was enthralled but also nervous. She was about to graduate from a small prestigious college in Texas. Her father was a successful business executive and decorated military commander in World War II. I was just the product of a lower middle-class home, graduate of a public university, and junior army officer.

But our cultural disparity did not bother her or her family. My family was a little intimidated, but greatly appreciated the burgeoning opportunities for service our familial connections would encourage.

Dad was right. It was the outwardly directed passion we shared that showed through everything else. We eventually created a plan for our lives together and pledged ourselves to do all we could to achieve the goals associated with that plan. Naturally, as the years sped by, the plan sometimes changed shape. But our fundamental beliefs and aspirations stayed the same.

Fast forward to the present.

Any legacy I leave is hers as well. Two magnificent sons who, because of their powers of discernment, married wonderful women. Three grandchildren who are all accomplished in their own ways. A church denomination that now encourages and celebrates the leadership of women. Public school students (especially women) who have grown into stable and contributing adults.

And public schools that are now structured to do a better job of comprehensively and authentically preparing students for a world of possibilities. All came from *our* passion to make a difference.

Alzheimer's Disease was not part of our plan. It has done more than just change the plan's shape. Eradicated is a better description. But the legacy remains.

A song from the movie *Camelot* reminds the viewer to not forget that for a brief moment there was a beautiful place called Camelot.

Camelot died because human passions went haywire. Our Camelot died because of Alzheimer's. But the memory of our mutually felt passion remains strong and somehow carries me through.

Chapter 3
Legacy

It is hard for me to think of myself as an octogenarian, albeit a "young" one. How can I have a wife who is eighty, who sits in a memory care facility unable to take care of her most basic needs?

Our *always* turned into a *legacy*, defined as something no longer eternal but what is left behind. The passion, once emanating from what "we" created over fifty-eight years, is now mine alone to sustain. Is it worth sustaining? Is it worth valuing?

If both of us died today at the same hour and minute, we would leave enough legacy. Our sons and grandchildren would collect the memorabilia, pictures, diplomas, certificates of accomplishment, and other leavings of a lifetime dedicated to service. Hopefully, those things would give comfort. A certainty that those of us who went before did more than live out our lives in purposeless and unproductive contentment.

Some people enjoy saying, "Life is what it is." Shoulders shrug as if to say there is not any real reason for our taking up space on this globe. We are no different than other mammals who eat, breathe, reproduce, and die.

It is what it is. Sigh.

But I do not agree with that assessment of our existence. I like to think human beings are an exceptional species with the talent, intelligence, and drive to create something approximating a Utopian environment. In addition, human beings are sentient creatures who can discern and therefore acknowledge a spiritual presence, one that envelopes us in the beauty and wonder of the universe.

Those of us who choose service as a way of life must ensure that every member of the species benefits from our actions. That they enjoy and grow from the power of nature, music, art, philosophy, religious beliefs and all other marvels of human achievement.

A spouse who remains after death or the advent of Alzheimer's, who was once a member of a married team dedicated to service, has the responsibility to keep the dream alive. Even now, while in the last stages of Alzheimer's, my wife will smile when I tell her about what I'm doing as a state AARP leader, or the author of a new book on school reform, or even my dabbling in writing this manuscript.

What I hope is registered behind that smile is that my current efforts and accomplishments are merely a preservation of what the two of us started together.

The AARP service is simply a continuation of studies and actions we took to support development of a university gerontology program in the 1970s. The school reform effort was a commonly felt passion in the late 1960s, out of which ideas, journal articles, and onsite service activities were spawned over decades. Even the writing of this book came from our determination to extend our influence through writing, workshops, and conference presentations.

True, we offered more individually initiated goals, such as my wife's dedication to helping church women assert leadership. And, as a terrific middle school science teacher, she inspired her female students. Many of them fondly remember her now.

I had little to do with those aspects of her service. But I did provide strong and ongoing support for her efforts. As I recount those achievements to her now, she smiles and looks contented.

Sometimes I wonder if end-of-life afflictions such as Alzheimer's leave any discernable legacy of their own. My wife has been a resident of a small memory care facility for over three years. Before the COVID–19 pandemic I visited her in that facility every day. I also met other residents, staff, and family visitors.

The symptoms of Alzheimer's and other forms of dementia manifest slowly and sometimes erratically. My wife and I were both educators, so the workings of the human brain interested us. It is a remarkable organ, even when it starts to misfire and shut down. As a husband, I was especially interested in how Alzheimer's affected the emotion of love.

I noticed visiting wives and husbands always try to elicit some sign that their afflicted spouse still loves them. With few exceptions, the resident will respond in some positive way and try to reciprocate.

It may be a cliché, but it seems clear to me that love remains long after most other parts of the brain and personality disappear. It is a kind of final legacy. After everything else fades away, the love remains and is transmitted to others in the only way possible.

Over the three years my wife has been in the facility I have created a picture album, a family memory notebook. When I or staff members guide my wife through its pages she often smiles, or her eyes flash a little. I am convinced that a memory was triggered somehow, emanating from feelings of her deep love of family members and the joy they brought to her life.

What a wonderful legacy for spouses and family members! After all the emotional pain caused by a disorder of the brain, the afflicted one is conveying love to everyone. She manifests that her life with them was worthwhile, even with this kind of ending.

In terms of my wife and our marital relationship it is important for my own mental and emotional balance that I discuss my relationship with Alzheimer's Disease. The legacy the disease leaves, by itself and in concert with social mores and expectations, is powerful.

I consider myself to be a responsible and moral man of eighty-two, thankfully blessed with comparatively good mental, emotional, and physical health. Yet my current life floats in a kind of twilight zone. I am a married man, but I must live alone, be alone, and continuously stay true to my vows. Month after month, year after year. Social interactions must be casual because any kind of intimacy, in whatever innocent form, is considered by folks from my era as disloyal.

I have become a little resentful about those perceptions. My resources ensure good care for my wife, and I am attentive to her and my family.

I am lucky. Other husbands and wives may shrivel because of one-on-one caregiving responsibilities within the home. They sometimes wither and die before the afflicted spouse does.

Wives often develop a helpful sisterhood. Men do not approach their buddies with a similar idea. At least, I don't.

How then, can we husbands explore and confront dementia?

Chapter 4
Loneliness

In my journey as an Alzheimer's caregiver, I am working through an emotional period characterized by a relationship schism. Death is not final, but its potential is mentally and emotionally omnipresent.

This is a strange kind of loneliness, somewhat different than what others suffer. That does not mean I am unique, but I think about it more than some. As an AARP state leader, I join my associates in studying loneliness, seeking ways it can be mitigated.

Loneliness has reached epidemic proportions. Health officials know this is not an idle observation but can be proven as a scientific fact. Loneliness is so severe it kills Americans at a rate equivalent to those who smoke fifteen cigarettes a day. It is so pervasive organizations such as AARP study it and support attempts to overcome it.

In 2020 we have lived with a viral pandemic, social unrest due to egregious past inequities, long simmering economic disparities growing into cultural disputes, and social support systems such as education in disarray. On the surface, all these disruptions to life may or may not be relevant to the loneliness epidemic. On the surface, our current turmoil is not directly related to the loneliness of a husband who cares for a wife with Alzheimer's.

But underneath the surface are treasured activities no longer safe in a pandemic: not being able to visit my wife at her facility, not interacting with the people who care for her, or not hosting family visits in which birthdays are celebrated and pictures taken.

Further under the surface are feelings of disorientation. Society seems to be unraveling. The possibility of a future quite different than anything my wife and I knew or remembered. What I considered to be *always*, *passion*, and *legacy* are now buried in a blurry present foreshadowed by an even less visible future.

That makes me feel even more lonely than before.

Where is that wife with whom I could share my fears and possible ways of dealing with a changing world? Together we worked our way through Cold War concerns and my possible military deployment in a major confrontation with what was then the USSR. Vietnam controversies, agitations of the 1960s, and other challenges ranged in scope from monumental to mundane.

In those days, with all their upheavals, I do not remember being lonely. Even if my wife and I were not physically together for a while, the relationship's aura was amazingly pervasive. It supported a feeling of confidence and tranquility as we wove our way through a life filled with amazing opportunities and challenges. My wife is still with us physically. But the "aura" is gone.

Other people, as nice as they are, cannot replace it. Governments, organizations like AARP, community senior centers, casinos, bingo parlors, country clubs, and retirement homes are not enough. Other attempts to make senior citizens comfortable and temporarily entertained or diverted do not work for me. Not even sports. Although religion always played a powerful role in my life, something is lacking there too.

Maybe it has something to do with a search for meaning. I vividly remember a time when my wife and I went out for ice cream while the kids were in school. Together we had achieved a milestone in terms of degree completion, and I had accepted a job in another state. Like many other couples in similar circumstances, we were both excited and nervous about the road ahead.

My wife said something strange, "I feel like my job is over."

During the previous ten years, the meaning of her life was to support me in my quest—to launch me in a direction I had always dreamed about.

She was an essential part of that effort. But until that moment I did not realize how tangential she felt her role was. The internal mechanism of the pact we made to serve education was working well, but her part of the deal up to that point was peripheral.

Now what? What was her new role in accomplishing our goals? She needed a better picture of what the meaning of our lives would be from that point forward.

Over bowls of ice cream, we adjusted our relationship and embellished on the original "service" reason for our union. We tweaked it. We defined its component parts. The whimsical meaning we once gave our allegiance became more defined and realistic.

More focused. More mutually supportive.

Now I crave that mutually supportive meaning. I long for another opportunity to eat ice cream together and search for a more definitive meaning for our union. But all I have left of that union is a legacy that does not exactly fit today's situation. All I can do is continue the search for meaning on my own.

My recently completed book on school reform, *The Teacher as Somebody*, should have meaning. But it was written before the pandemic and social unrest. Does it have meaning now?

An AARP project to help both young and old rethink the meaning of aging is in development. But it has to be instituted virtually. Will that work?

My little church gives me emotional and spiritual support, but the pastor and wonderful members of the congregation are not always able to help me find the kind of meaning I am looking for. How could they? They want to love me like I love them as Christian brothers and sisters. But their milieu is not mine.

Some can only imagine what my caregiving situation is like. Few of them can share the type or level of meaning my wife and I subscribed to. But I appreciate their thoughts and prayers.

As a man accustomed to ongoing engagement with my wife and others committed to changing the status quo in education, aloneness does not appeal to me.

My thoughts twist around the difference between loneliness and a variation of aloneness.

Chapter 5
Aloneness

In March of 1962, I had a third date with a college senior. While third dates are not uncommon, our dates involved my driving five hours from central Texas to near the Oklahoma border. My military obligations were demanding, and time off was precious, so I must have been captivated by this young woman.

But on that third date I began to wonder—was I being smart about this budding relationship? She revealed a side of herself I was not sure I could handle. Over a restaurant dinner she told me how much she loved to dance. Me? I could take it or leave it.

Every noon hour she and her friends danced to the jukebox at the student union. She told me about some of the young men who participated in that early afternoon tea dance.

During my weekend visits I stayed overnight in a men's dorm. So I had met two or three of these guys. They seemed nice. My date told me at least one of them was homosexual. And she had become his confidant and friend. She made it clear that her own preferences were not in any way similar. But she cared for this gentle pre-ministerial major who was suffering psychologically, spiritually, and emotionally. It was 1962, after all, and attitudes then were quite different than today.

I listened.

Given the era, I was not sure what to think about this young woman. She was willing to counsel a man who, in my military unit, would be cashiered out as soon as possible. My church called his condition a sin. In polite society he would have been considered a pariah. For him to even consider the ministry was ludicrous.

The woman I was dating lived in a dormitory with female students who could not understand why she would befriend this man. And I, too, had a difficult time coming to grips with it.

I left that weekend making no plans to return. "I'll stay in touch," I muttered noncommittally. She made no effort to encourage my return.

The drive back seemed much longer than five hours. I felt conflicted. By the time I drove into the post I was emotionally exhausted. The subsequent days and weeks were filled with difficult and dangerous military maneuvers and exercises. But I was almost grateful for them as I could focus on the danger rather than this woman.

This situation was not something I wanted to discuss with my fellow officers. I am certain they would have told me, "Walk away. There are other fish in the sea."

So I felt alone as I mulled over the issues. And in my aloneness, I grasped a few revelations.

What kind of woman was I dating? No doubt, she met my father's description of someone with substance and conviction. Her convictions were scripturally based—to love others even if the guy was in fact a sinner.

How alone he must feel, especially if his sin was something he could not help because of biological and psychological wiring. How alone my young woman must feel when risking the friendship of both male and female students on campus.

I sensed she liked me. What courage it took to share with me a story that was so counterculture. Was she testing me? Maybe. Could I develop her kind of courage? I did not think so.

But slowly my admiration of her grew. Many women I dated up to that point were self-absorbed and superficially judgmental of others. I could not think of even one who would reach out to someone in need, much less risk the prejudicial opinion of their peers. They sought social acceptance, often through membership in a college sorority. My young woman was not interested in that kind of status.

I sensed she wanted my love, but only if she could be an authentic Christian servant to those shunned or held at arm's length. Our discussions about what she wished to accomplish in education clearly brought out those points.

She risked the possibility of being alone the rest of her life if her prospective mate could not accept who and what she was as a caring woman. As a human being who both wanted and needed meaning in her life.

One night I wrote her a long letter. Apologies. You know, intense military training and all that. I asked for another weekend date. She wrote back. "No need for an apology." She would be pleased to see me again.

A few months later we were married. And for nearly fifty-eight years she has reached out to others less fortunate or shunned. Her students. People in the churches to which we belonged. Others who needed to know they were not alone and rejected.

A life well lived! Even now, within the fog of Alzheimer's.

Aloneness is much different than feeling lonely. That college senior I dated taught me much about the importance of holding well-reasoned and valid convictions in the face of possible rejection.

No, it has not been an Ayn Rand story such as *The Fountainhead*, in which the hero remains an individual true to his own talents in the face of overwhelming rejection. It is instead the acceptance of the Christian credo that we stand by the "least of these." No matter what. No matter how much we are disdained, shunned, or criticized for breaking any social standard now in vogue.

Aloneness is often the result of living or working outside the lines of social expectations. It was more palatable when "I" was part of a "we." Pillow talk. Coffee in the morning. Solace in the face of what seemed like insurmountable odds.

Old habits are hard to break even when the "we" is absorbed by Alzheimer's. Aloneness, therefore, is more agonizing than ordinary loneliness.

Chapter 6
Engagement

To find enough meaning in my life, I must be engaged in something. I need to interact with other people. And the interaction must have a certain dynamic, a kind of vigorous back and forth. To the extent that happens, my feelings of aloneness dissipate. My wife and I could do that without resorting to anger. Until her dementia interfered.

It took a while for me to realize what was happening. What we once enjoyed as productive banter became more like arguing. No meeting of the minds anymore. Our pledge to never go to bed angry with one another was getting harder to fulfill.

Even before admitting my wife to a residential care facility, I sensed aloneness. The kind of electric spark that once connected us psychically, was weakening. What happened to it? Was it me? Where was the congruence we experienced eating ice cream and planning the future? How could I get that kind of engagement back?

Slowly, even agonizingly, I realized I could not.

At that point I began to define aloneness as a lack of dynamic engagement with someone (or people) with whom I had formed an essential bond.

Biologists report that feelings of loneliness are normal defense mechanisms emanating from our primeval past. Like all mammals, our ancestors knew that being alone for any length of time could be fatal. The herd provides safety. Protection from the saber-toothed tiger lurking outside the group of humans circled around the fire.

Feelings of aloneness come from a higher plain of existence than mere survival. For example, some of my military colleagues "re-upped" because the army became their family. They loved the camaraderie, esprit de corps, and even the "one for all and all for one" associated with the three musketeers.

I remember an older-than-usual captain with whom I served in the army. During World War II he was a first sergeant, but after discharge he was reduced to selling vacuum cleaners door-to-door. He descended from a position of authority in a magnificent cause to a guy selling cleaning equipment to housewives.

He felt alone and sidelined from life. While not easy, he returned to the army, attended OCS just before his twenty-eighth birthday, and became a "regular." Even with severe PTSD from horrific war experiences, and pervasive insomnia, he was happier than when he walked alone from house to house.

For forty-three years I was a professor and consultant to public schools throughout the nation. Much of that time my wife was my "sidekick"—the result of our ice cream compact. Together we hosted special classes in our home, co-authored articles, and worked in state and national associations.

We prepared for and traveled to dozens of workshops and association conferences. We socialized with local faculty members and made friendships throughout the country. We were also active in our church and the activities of our sons.

We were fully engaged with each other and the world around us. We never experienced aloneness, even when my wife had to leave for weeks on end to take care of infirmed parents in another state. That was just temporary separation.

The aura remained.

A difference exists between what I call "intense engagement" and ordinary engagement. That distinction does not resonate with most people, but it certainly does with me. So this may be where my story becomes more anomaly than commonplace.

My wife understood my tendency to be dubious. She also understood that it was, and still is, difficult for me to blithely accept something as fact if I think the "context" is insufficient. In other words, I can be a hard sell. Some might call me a pain in the neck.

Before joining a university faculty, I taught secondary school history and government. Although never a debater myself, I liked debate's insistence on supporting opinion with facts. Therefore, I used the process as a teaching method in grades six through twelve.

In a debate, no statement is considered sacrosanct. Everything said is subject to questioning and an insistence on seeing or hearing evidence. While many people today find that process annoying, it is nevertheless the cornerstone of a fully functioning democracy. And I believe in it! So, what does that personality quirk of mine have to do with *Confronting Dementia*?

Remember the story I related about how my "date" supported a homosexual man while in college? My first inclination was to ignore the context and accept prevailing prejudices. I was ready to dismiss any woman who would associate with that "kind" of person. In 1962 terms the evidence was egregious.

But what my future wife taught me is that evidence can turn against itself, if considered in the light of compassion, love, and a drive to lift humanity as God expects. She taught me that evidence and context must be painted with a broader brush. She introduced me to the literary works of C. S. Lewis, many of which she studied in classes at her church-related college. While I had heard of that world-renowned scholar, I did not know much about him or his view of the world.

My wife said, "Understanding Lewis is not easy. He struggled to understand who and what he was in the context of faith, theologically based evidence, and different interpretations of words and language in general."

He had been traumatized by the early death of his mother and experiences on the front lines of World War I. He became a dedicated atheist convinced that no loving God would ever allow so much human suffering. Lewis was complex and dubious about everything. That never changed. What did change was his understanding, and ultimate belief in Christianity. His was not a dramatic conversion. In some ways it was not a conversion at all. It was, instead, a continuing engagement with historical context, pros and cons, and an ongoing evaluation of evidence and the meaning of truth.

I understand his struggle. And I understand what Lewis endured with the suffering and death of his wife. Those events were instructive to him and caused him to become more engaged with life than ever.

Perhaps his understanding of truth might help with my need for engagement.

Chapter 7
Faith

I envy people who can accept faith as a given. For them, belief in God and the spiritual world either is or is not. And the "is not" requires no consideration at all.

The power of prayer cannot be debated. Intellectualizing the meaning of Christ's life and death on the cross is unacceptable. Scripture is to be read and discussed to achieve better understanding of meaning, and how that meaning translates into our behavior and depth of faith. A plethora of writers and leaders can explain what that meaning is or should be.

Everything about this belief system is based on deductive reasoning. The words are inviolable because they are God's message to us. It is blasphemous to think otherwise. Thus, people who blaspheme are to be pitied and prayed for, lest they fall into depravity. They are transgressors who are a danger to themselves and others.

Absolutes. Inescapable truisms. The need to subjugate one's own will to that of the Lord. Acceptance of a spiritual world typically referred to as a kingdom, with a benevolent God who expects all of us to follow his guidance without questioning his authority. Thy will be done.

C.S. Lewis approached the topic of faith as an inductive thinker. In nearly all his books on faith and religion, everything tended to percolate up. As depicted in the movie biopic of his life, *Shadowlands*, he struggled with the topics of suffering and grief. In short, he could intellectualize God's will regarding the purpose and value of human despair. But faced with suffering and grief in the highly personal experience associated with the illness and death of his wife, his theorizing unraveled.

Lewis had been down that road before with the death of his mother and another woman with whom he felt a special closeness. Those events shook him to the core. But it was the illness and death of his beloved wife that tested his faith almost to the limit.

Intellectualizing loss, grief, and the role of God in our lives did not protect Lewis any more than it protects me from my wife's Alzheimer's journey. But try as I might, switching from inductive to deductive faith is not working very well either. I still cannot shift my faith to an unbounded "thy will be done," or the "it is what it is" phrase so popular today.

How can a husband view faith as a solace for overcoming unremittent sadness and grief? In trying to answer that question, I wonder what the phrase, "We are praying for you" means to those who say it and those who hear it.

I admit to being a kind of C. S. Lewis Christian, one who understands how words and phrases can be interpreted to create a highly personal kind of Christ-centered faith. While nowhere nearly as insightful or intelligent as Lewis was, I can identify with his search for linguistic meaning. In *Mere Christianity* for example.

I may have stumbled through an ecclesiastical minefield, a venture with the potential to offend or be misunderstood. I do not want any reader to think I am insensitive to the love and caring of friends, members of a church congregation, or any other devout believers who honestly and sincerely seek to offer me comfort.

I feel the depth of their spirit-based empathy and appreciate it. Their motives and love for me are never in doubt. But the phrase, "we are praying for you" tends to fall into an emotional vacuum.

It is hard to explain why. Individuals and groups will refer to me by name in sincere and beautifully articulated prayers. They will ask that I be comforted. They request that my wife be shielded from pain and distress as she navigates the stormy waters of progressive dementia.

This is called "intercessory prayer." It is thought to be especially powerful because the prayer is lifted up by many in my name and on behalf of my wife.

Many churches, including my own, systematize it through use of prayer lists. Communal activities carefully and prayerfully ensure that no one is overlooked. They ensure that ongoing circumstances such as ours are always uppermost in their minds.

When I am told I am being "prayed for," I know it is true and it is authentic. It is believed to be powerful. And I love the people who participate because they want me to be comforted as much as possible.

So does my problem mean I am a man of little faith? Am I a cynic? Is my status as a Christian questionable? Would "We are thinking of you" be any better? Probably not, although I treasure the sentiment in the same way I appreciate condolences when a loved one dies. "They mean well" is the usual explanation. And I know they do.

My problem goes back to the topic of engagement. When a condolence or expression of prayerful concern is clearly heartfelt enough for me to feel it both emotionally and spiritually. Deep down. With unmitigated love woven into it.

When the other person or persons somehow convey a deep connection with me, an enveloping sensation stays with me for hours, even days. The other person's prayers may not necessarily be articulate or part of a systematic process. But they strike me as being expressions of deep Christian empathy and a oneness of the spirit. Our souls have become spiritually engaged. How significant that connection is with me! It pervades my thoughts and emotions.

It can also be dangerous in the context of giving it a meaning that does not or should not exist. It must not have *anything* to do with carnality or personal attraction. It takes maturity on the part of both the recipient of the caring remark and the one who offers it unguardedly, to keep it in the realm of authentic, moral, and lasting comfort.

Chapter 8
Gender

As a state volunteer for AARP, I have been identified as particularly interested in problems associated with caregiving. Since so much of today's caregiving service revolves around some form and degree of dementia, my "specialty," is concentrated on that subject. This categorization feels uncomfortable, because I am no longer an in-home caregiver.

As a careful financial planner, I have prepared for my wife's needs. She is now in an exceptional memory care facility. It features a homelike atmosphere in which only eight residents each have their own room. The facility is fully staffed with competent individuals who maintain a family atmosphere and are supported by highly qualified medical personnel.

The configuration of a man taking care of his wife is not the prevailing narrative. I read and attend conferences on caregiving for Alzheimer's patients. The stories are typically about a woman taking care of a parent, grandparent, or husband. Even the narrative of a wife taking care of a husband is not especially common.

Over the past three years I have met many caregivers. Some have become my friends. Before the pandemic we often chatted. We got to know each other and shared about our lives prior to and at the onset of our loved ones' dementia. Most of our stories were variations on a central theme. Occasionally we had lunch together.

Regarding Alzheimer's and caregiving in general, does gender matter? As with most distinctions in life, it depends on cultural habits, beliefs, and mores. It also depends on the norms of a particular era and how we view divisions of labor.

Today's cultural norm is one reason I decided to write this book. My intent is not to suggest that my emotional and attitudinal struggles are symbolic of the way all husbands feel. To do that I would need to conduct research across a broad spectrum of men in the population who care for afflicted wives.

The subjects of my research would be separated into various classifications: education, occupation, profession, financial standing, or age. I would include an examination of other involvements that have the potential for influencing behaviors and the ability to handle responsibility and stress.

I will leave that endeavor to someone younger and more capable. In fact, someone may be already studying the situation.

As much as possible, I want to avoid hackneyed stereotypes:

- That women are the nurturing sex and therefore wired to be sensitive to the needs of others.
- That women tend to be more loving and interested in ministering to those in pain and emotional distress.
- That women are more willing to help loved ones who can no longer perform basic tasks such as showering or using the toilet.

Most men want to avoid worrying about ADL (activities of daily living). I know I do.

Some women are terrible caregivers. Some men are good caregivers. Both men and women provide excellent care for their spouses without *giving evidence* of being severely affected emotionally, physically, or spiritually. I know many of these caregivers.

The ill effects of caregiving are not always clearly seen. Sometimes a little digging below the surface reveals problems they cover up. Until they cannot.

Case in point: a friend called to tell me our mutual friends were in deep trouble. This couple is financially secure. The wife has declined cognitively for years. Her husband refuses to accept help from friends. They have no children, nor do they have family members close to them. Just a small social group that includes people their age who have problems of their own.

The wife's behavior is bizarre, and rational conversation is not possible. The husband, once a man of average build, now weighs about 100 pounds. Determined to continue taking care of his wife.

My suggestion was to call the help line of the local Alzheimer's Association as soon as possible. Without intervention, the situation will reach a resolution involving emergency medical services and perhaps, police involvement.

Many years ago, this couple lived in our neighborhood. I did not know them well. As far as I knew, the husband was quiet, somewhat distant, loyal and a hard-working success, at least in terms of making money and taking care of his wife. The wife was a teacher with a network of friends until they moved to a more affluent neighborhood. By that time, she was losing her ability to speak and be rational. Too late.

What would have happened if conditions were different, if the husband had become afflicted instead? If they did not move away from a previously supportive community? So many "ifs." If the wife had made the decisions, become the caregiver, and talked openly with her friends, I think the outcome would have been different. No way of knowing for sure.

It does not take mounds of data to support the observation that women are often part of a supportive sisterhood. The existence of a nearby family, or at least a community of mutually supportive friends, can make a big difference. And women are more inclined to take advantage of that available assistance.

My wife and I discussed contingencies. We worked together to prepare for the future. Many of my male friends would rather pretend everything will be fine forever. They will someday pay a price either as the caregiver or the afflicted one.

So, our finances were in order. We lived close to reliable medical services. We maintained the already solid relationship with our extended family. We explored housing options and maintained our membership in a supportive church.

Maybe gender is less a consideration than planning together. It was for us.

Chapter 9
Relationships

If you want someone to sleep with during cold, lonely nights, adopt a dog or a cat. Not all men or women agree. Some do not like animals in the house and certainly, not in bed with them.

My wife loves animals, so for many years we had either a dog or a cat sleeping with us. In the memory care home in which she now lives, they have a resident cat. When Facebook pictures are shared, my wife is often cuddling the kitten. In one video clip she is shown kissing it. Sweet.

Except for rare occasions when I keep my granddaughter's cat, I have no animal in my retirement villa. Sometimes I am tempted to get one. For now, my solace at night is a little Bose radio hooked to Sirius XM, a satellite service most often used in automobiles. I cannot tolerate most of the stations, but it does carry soft instrumental music which I find relaxing at a low volume. My wife and I agreed to never install a TV in the bedroom. Specialists in sleep disorders report this is a good idea. So I perpetuate the practice.

Even during this time of supposedly enlightened thinking, relationships are culturally proscribed for people of certain genders, ages, cultural affiliations, religions, and socio-economic levels. Stereotypes abound. A few rock-solid regulations exist, but there is an undercurrent of what is considered socially acceptable or not.

I have always valued the importance of a religious and moral life. In some ways I may be far from typical. For now, I am caught in my own cultural stereotype.

Our years of marriage are admired by others. The ongoing love felt for my wife and two sons is personally satisfying. My sons are my best friends and enormously supportive in more ways than I can count. I have terrific friends, professional colleagues, and congenial neighbors. My life has been and continues to be rich and full. The fact I am healthy, with a brain that still functions fairly well, is in some ways surprising to me. My brain continues to allow me to interact with the world. That is no longer the case with my wife, the other half of *me* for over half a century.

The carryover from our "we" years is all encompassing. During that time we developed a worldview that amalgamated the spiritual with the rational. We mixed our belief in Christian teachings with secular (practical) ideas.

Everything we prayed about or reflected on in a spiritual way needed real life context. And our personal and professional behaviors were designed to reflect that perspective. It was the essence of our dedication to service.

Pillow talk. Both of us discussed what this time of our lives might be like. We knew one of us would need to finish an existence in this world without the other. That time arrived unexpectedly, but a variation on a theme.

The theme is pending death. The variation is Alzheimer's.

Sometimes natural or spiritual metaphors are a kind of relationship unto themselves. They have personalities and a type of ethereal substance. They may seem to replace the missing part of the loved one who is slowly fading away. I cannot achieve that kind of reflective writing.

Is it the "male" in me? Am I deficient in spiritual depth?

A thread of "always" or "legacy" completes the memory of what my wife once was and, in some ways, continues to be. But it is not spiritual for me. I can think of no metaphors that fill in the empty spaces like pieces in a jigsaw puzzle.

Although I tend to be an academic with a moral compass, one who probably thinks and writes too much, I am still biologically human. I often long for what was. Yet sometimes I wonder if the "what was" can be replicated in someone else. Not a facsimile of my wife. Not a romantic involvement.

Just someone sitting across the room or table from me, encouraging me one moment, and telling me how wrong I am the next. Not just a sounding board. Certainly not an alter ego or soul mate. Perhaps a confidant, someone I can trust with my innermost thoughts and beliefs.

For some reason I am unable to think of that person as a buddy, another man. I enjoy being with guys my age, but not in that engaging way. We talk about the usual stuff: cars, politics, sports, travel, adventure, business, money, and property. Occasionally the conversation turns slightly more personal, but we avoid touchy-feely topics like the plague. The sisterhood of women at least partially overcomes that problem. I envy them.

For me, during this twilight zone in which I am living, personal conversations with a woman are seen as socially off-kilter. I am a married man. There is something disloyal about getting too far into certain topics with a woman who is not my wife.

I do not pretend to be in any way symbolic of most men in my situation—or even in similar caregiving circumstances. All human beings are different, and men are no exception.

Chapter 10
You

Caregiving stories are everywhere, and many defy classification. This book is not just about me, or even "we." I do not consider myself symbolic of men who become caregivers. My story does not include poverty, collapsing societies, intercultural warfare, or other disruptions that impinge on every decision. Every action. That knowledge humbles me. It makes my story seem almost trivial.

The contributions of women as mothers, daughters, wives, and caring members of an extended family or community impress me. I have met many of you. At my wife's memory care home. In my neighborhood, church, and online. For almost sixty years I worked with you as schoolteachers, students, as team members on campus and in the consultant field. I met you at national associations and as a supporter of my wife's efforts to improve the quality of women's lives everywhere. Your stories are filled with dedication and selfless service. Now I see you as nurses and caregivers working diligently to care for those afflicted with the COVID–19 virus.

My writing coach told me that my writing should connect with readers. My work with AARP and other groups gave me clues. But was that enough?

Many of you have more important stories than mine. So I have sought those stories and polished them a little. Then used the medium of blogging and book compilation to inform and inspire others.

Below are a few classifications that might resonate with my readers. I call them fictitious scenario snippets.

Real Men are Not Whiners: Life has its ups and downs, but I am emotionally strong. I do not complain or seek help from others. I can take care of myself. And I can certainly take care of my wife.

If health and financial concerns arise during our life together, I will solve them myself. I have been a good provider and problem solver, always there when my wife needed help or guidance. Thanks for your offer of assistance, but no thanks. I can take care of my wife's decline by myself.

Success in Life is Multifaceted: I have been successful in business, and my family has benefited from it. Achieving success in anything is mostly a matter of staying informed, acting when the situation calls for it, and building support networks.

While I admit that my wife's dementia is a different kind of challenge, a cursory review of available services reveals many organizations I can engage. My wife's dementia is irreversible and will eventually result in her death. Our adult children are busy with their own lives and reside in another state, but I hope they understand the situation with their mother and visit her occasionally. In the meantime, I plan to stay active with my business pursuits and my golf game.

God Is Ever Present in Our Lives: My wife and I have been active church-goers our entire married life. We are devout Christians and believe in the saving grace of our Lord Jesus Christ. We believe unerringly that Jesus died on the cross to save us from our sins. Scripture tells us life on earth was never meant to be easy, but we will achieve everlasting life in heaven.

This truth helps me endure my wife's Alzheimer's journey, because I know she will eventually die from its effects. Sometimes I worry that her excruciatingly long decline to inevitable death is my fault, possibly the penance we must make for some sin I committed. Sometimes I cry when no one else is looking. And I constantly seek forgiveness.

Marriage is a Necessary Burden: Marriage has been historically considered either an economic or political necessity. Peasants married to produce children who could help with farm work or otherwise contribute to a family's income. Ruling classes married to improve a nation state's allegiances and trade alliances and to produce heirs to the family dynasty.

Even in today's America, marriage (or co-habitation) is seen by some as a practical way of life. In some ways that reasoning was the foundation of our marriage which has lasted decades.

But now I am confused because my wife is dying of Alzheimer's. Each day she fades away a little more. The practicality of marriage has evolved into something else. What for years was nothing more than a convenient arrangement for us is now turning into something quite different. It affects my psyche and emotions. And it scares me. What will I do without her? Who will I be when she is gone?

Institutionalization is Unacceptable: Everyone knows that growing old in your own home and neighborhood is better than being placed in some institution. A blissful old age is touted as being one in which you die in your own bed, in the home you love, surrounded by members of your family.

My wife and I often talked about this scenario. It was her wish. She never made me promise to help her achieve that goal, but it was certainly implied. Even after the diagnosis of Alzheimer's, I diligently tried to keep my wife home. And for years I did it.

Until she became a danger to both herself and me. Until she wandered down the street in the middle of the night. Until she forgot how to get dressed, take a shower, or use the toilet. Until I was coming apart emotionally and physically because of stress.

Signing the contract for her to be admitted to a memory care facility was like signing a death warrant. And I cried every time she called and said, "I'm ready to come home now."

Chapter 11
Scenarios

The following fictitious scenarios of husbands taking care of their wives still ring with an aura of truth. They are based on real life stories. While some negative situations might have been handled differently, what the husband did may simply be a good response to the challenge of Alzheimer's or another form of dementia.

Too Young, Too Soon, Too Burdensome: My wife is only fifty-three. We have been married over thirty years. Our three children are now adults. So far, they have given us two grandchildren. Our two married daughters live in a nearby town. Our youngest, a son, still lives at home while attending graduate school at the local university.

At fifty-five, I still work as an engineer in a local manufacturing plant. My wife works part time as a secretary at a local law office. About a year ago my wife's employer called to ask if I had noticed anything different about my wife's behavior.

"A little, I guess. She gets more confused than usual and seems somewhat more depressed."

The employer said she had noticed the same thing. "It's getting to be a problem at work. I suggest you seek a medical opinion ... a good physical."

We visited our primary care physician who referred us to a neurologist. Tests were conducted. They eliminated treatable conditions such as hormonal disorders, an infection, or the aftereffects of a mild stroke. The diagnosis was early onset dementia which further tests indicated was probably Alzheimer's Syndrome.

Devastating news. There is no way to predict how rapidly the situation would worsen. But plans must be made by the family. Her job. My job. Finances. Travel modifications. Eventual in-home care. Possible future institutionalization. Long-term care insurance.

Now I cannot stand watching all the TV ads showing happy seniors living out their "golden years" in some retirement wonderland. What am I going to do now?

PTSD Multiplied: I am a veteran with two tours of duty in Vietnam with the Marines. Now at seventy, I am semi-retired from various kinds of employment, mostly in construction. While I was only slightly wounded in Vietnam, the experiences in firefights and their aftermath left me shaken. Despair. Anger. Suicidal tendencies. Substance abuse. Broken relationships. Even homelessness for a short time. I went through two marriages that produced three children, but they ended in divorce. My adult kids want nothing to do with me.

Six years ago, I met a wonderful woman who accepted me with all my faults. We married. She has endured much in our relationship: fights with the Veterans Administration, hospitalizations, treatment centers, nightmares, bizarre behaviors, financial problems.

I love her and depend on her, try to show my gratitude. She is my everything. Two years ago, she was diagnosed with Alzheimer's. We try to take care of each other and have a few friends who help when they can. Our future will likely involve becoming wards of the state. That means we will be separated. I would rather die.

Follow the Money: Because my wife and I both have pre-existing conditions, purchasing any kind of life or long-term care insurance has been either impossible or a frustrating challenge. As responsible and hard-working citizens, neither of us want to live in a cradle-to-grave socialist country. We accept the economic philosophy of free enterprise.

On the other hand, we dread the future. I am still two years away from qualifying for Medicare. Because of a disability my wife does not work outside the home. At age sixty-three, I could start collecting minimal Social Security payments even while keeping my job as an HVAC repair technician. But waiting two or perhaps seven years will substantially increase our monthly payments.

Our doctor says my wife is showing early signs of dementia, and family history suggests the possibility of Alzheimer's. As we study the situation, we find little reason for hope. With help from family members, I can forestall retirement two years. Medicare, Social Security, and any part time work I do will allow me to take care of my wife at home.

However, if anything happens to me as my wife requires institutional care, the only option we have available is Medicaid. Its income and estate rules are severe. One of our daughters has begun exploring a movement called Dementia Friendly America. That possibility, along with the work of the Alzheimer's Association, AARP and others may not help people of modest means such as our family.

But it helps to think about the possibilities.

Chapter 12
Mike

My name is Mike. My wife's name is Karen. This is a story I wish I did not need to tell.

I am tired of hearing about Tevye, the main character in the Broadway play and 1971 movie titled *Fiddler on the Roof*. Karen bought the DVD of the movie and watched it regularly. A little too much, in my opinion.

Its storyline and music are creative and entertaining. But not so much after repeated showings. When Karen pulled the DVD off the closet shelf, I would get scarce. Yard work. Walk the dog. Retreat to the kitchen and read one of my Tom Clancy novels. Maybe a nap somewhere in the house where I did not have to listen to the lyrics of "If I Were a Rich Man."

After the DVD ended Karen would find me. She would say, "You know, you're an awful lot like Tevye."

I would always ask, "How?"

"Because you're stuck in an attitudinal culture just as much as he is."

"Attitudinal culture? Now that is an interesting turn of phrase."

"Well, you are! You do not come from the culture in which the fictional Tevye was born. But in some ways your experiences were similar. Those experiences you had in your family and community rubbed off on you."

"Here we go again."

Eventually we would get to the heart of it. According to Karen, I am a 1950s male traditionalist. In those years superheroes were men who protected the weak and innocent. Cowboy movie stars were either loners or accompanied only by their horses and sidekicks. Women in their lives, at the end of each movie, watched with tears in their eyes as the hero rode off into the sunset. The end.

Karen said real life is more complicated than Superman's motto of "Truth, Justice and the American Way." The arbiters of all three of those lofty goals were men. Traditional, God-fearing men. Men who took good care of the "little woman" and their offspring. Virtuous men who were willing to make sacrifices to care for and protect those they love.

Then came the word "suffocating." Karen explained how she greatly appreciated the continuing effort I made to ensure she and the family were well cared for. She loved me for it.

"But do you ever think of me as a real person? A true partner in life? You say you do, but never include me in discussions about substantive matters, like finances or making important decisions concerning our future direction. You insist you know best, that everything has been thought out carefully and planned for. I'm not to worry. But I do worry. And I feel marginalized, not valued."

I am not an idiot. There is truth in what Karen said. We often discussed our children, and I deferred to her opinion on that topic most of the time. But I know I dominated her in other ways, somewhat like my father:

- Property and job decisions
- Management of money
- Which car to buy
- What church to attend
- How to believe politically and who to vote for
- Even how we would spend vacations and when to visit relatives

As we grew older both of us started having health problems. That was expected. Because of a few bad experiences with the medical community and insurance companies, I let my opinion reign supreme. It was almost a compulsion on my part, so Karen held back. She let me be in control. After all, I did the research on the best options, so I made the decisions.

As the years rolled by Karen stopped using the word "suffocating." The word for her new behavior was more like "reticent." She quietly gave in to my opinion. At that stage in our lives there was no changing the dynamic of our relationship. I prevailed and she submitted.

Strangely though, I felt a growing sadness. Not a victorious elation. The more she submitted to my wishes, the more depressed I became.

I had a couple of small medical emergencies. Karen, with the help of our children, supported my treatment and recuperation. The children and I did the same for her when she had problems. But it was almost like sleepwalking through the days. We did what was expected.

Then Karen started to forget how to do things she had done all her life. Mostly small things at first. The doctor checked her blood pressure, potassium levels, and conducted other standard examinations of possible ordinary reasons for mild brain dysfunction. All were negative.

"It could be the onset of dementia," she said. "It can't be diagnosed definitively, so please bring her back every three months for follow-up evaluations. In the meantime, I'll prescribe a drug that is supposed to slow down the syndrome's progress."

And so, it began. A roller coaster ride at first, then a gradual shut-down. The odd feeling of sadness I felt earlier escalated into a full-blown depression. How could this be?

Real men do not whine!

I was always able to take care of my wife before. What was happening to me? Lack of sleep? Having to prepare meals? Cleaning up after accidents? Making excuses for Karen's occasional bizarre behaviors or strange comments?

My nights were spent wondering if the woman next to me was really Karen. If so, maybe I should apologize for the years I marginalized her, made her feel devalued as a human being and my partner in life. But then the morning's reality hits me with yet another crisis—another penance for years of acting like a jerk.

No escape. I needed help. At first our children and I made plans for in-home care. We searched for a suitable memory care facility—for later, when the time came.

No re-doing what was done in years past. Now I just dread the future.

Chapter 13
Don

My name is Don, and Susan is my wife. This story is about priorities and lives gone awry. Like Mike in the previous story, I am a product of mid-twentieth century America. My priorities were shaped by multifaceted experiences and beliefs.

Think Vietnam and the late 1960s:

- draft card burning
- antiwar demonstrations
- rock concerts
- Volkswagen Minivans painted in outrageous colors
- illegal drug use
- aimlessness
- bizarre behaviors
- anti-establishment rantings
- and lots of long hair

Susan and I met in high school. We were both from prominent well-to-do families. We were spoiled, with feelings of entitlement. We knew privilege. We were both gifted enough to be accepted by the best universities. Susan majored in international relations while I was pre-law.

Life for us looked promising and secure. But every night we saw disturbing events on our TV sets. Berkley demonstrations. Chicago riots during the democratic convention. The Woodstock phenomenon. Kent State shooting deaths. And more. It seemed as if our world were unraveling. Only my college deferment kept me from being tapped on the shoulder as the next soldier to die in Vietnam.

The military draft ended midway through my time in law school. By that time Susan and I had participated in some of the wild stuff, but kind of on the periphery. A couple of rock concerts. Some small demonstrations. Letters to the editor. No drugs or other excesses. We survived the maelstrom unscathed. Our kind of normal could be pursued as originally planned.

Stay on track. Maintain tight control. Do not rock the boat. Prepare for the unexpected, but be as ready for it as possible. Healthy eating and plenty of exercise. Even before our wedding, we were serious about financial planning. Investments. Insurance. Staying in close touch with our extended family and network of friends was a big part of our future.

We became politically active. But true to our station in life, we valued social stability over radical change. *Messy* does not work for those of us following the trajectory of success in life.

Susan and I married after I finished law school. She had completed her undergraduate work. But she decided her chosen field of international relations would involve too much travel and stress. She would be a stay-at-home wife and mother. I was grateful. With a specialty in corporate law, it was logical for me to become part of the business community. Not overly exciting, but stable and lucrative enough.

Stereotypically, we purchased a nice home in a comfortable upper middle-class neighborhood. We joined a country club, worked with our kids' schools as supporters and sponsors of various events. We found a church suitable for our beliefs which offered excellent programs for children and young people.

Susan did not work outside the home. I had a job with enough flexibility to take nice summer vacations. We enjoyed family travel throughout the nation and even certain spots in the world. Cruises. Disneyworld. Europe.

We gave money to good causes, and Susan participated in various kinds of charity work. Together we attended my professional conferences whenever possible. The American dream.

With few exceptions, our kids grew up with minimal health concerns and did well in school. Susan and I marched through occasional but treatable health problems. Minor inconveniences. Like everyone, we lost members of our extended families. Hospital visits. Care facilities. Funerals.

Susan and her mother were emotionally close. One day her mother, 79, fell and broke a hip, gashed her head. She was already suffering from COPD and other cardiopulmonary problems. I had never seen my wife fall apart. Her mother's physical condition improved slightly but cognitive abilities took a nosedive. As her mother's condition worsened, Susan became more depressed and anxious. Nothing I said or did seemed to help.

For years, our lives had been pleasant and uneventful. But now Susan was not able to control the anxiety over her mother.

Then I had a mild stroke on the golf course. EMTs were efficient and able to take me to an emergency room quickly enough to mitigate lasting damage. While I was not concerned about my problem, Susan was. She hovered over me. It almost drove me to distraction. Our relationship, once so warm and mutually sustaining, became fractured.

At least the events of the 1960s were external to our lives. Those challenges were "out there someplace." But the current multifaceted concerns were inside us. Almost impossible to control.

Finally, with my insistence, Susan sought counseling Everything improved a little until our youngest daughter was diagnosed with breast cancer. It was treatable, but Susan's emotional progress came to a screeching halt.

Walking the dog was an outlet for me. It got me out of the house. Out of the lunacy. I spent more time at the office and on the golf course.

Susan's mother died and our daughter's cancer was caught in time. The prognosis was good. But Susan became more depressed, out-of-touch with reality as she approached seventy. Her mother's accident and subsequent illnesses seemed to have triggered something in Susan's personality. Her driving was so erratic she received traffic tickets, something that never happened before. Friends drifted away.

Even our kids no longer enjoyed visiting us. Our once immaculate house became a mess, with the constant importation of stuffed animals, trinkets, and other odds and ends.

Any complaint from me about her behaviors sent Susan into a rage. She screamed, "You've always been selfish and uncaring. You never loved me."

Our life together was a dismal failure.

Thanks to a benevolent employer, I opted to work part-time beyond the usual retirement years. More time on the golf course. More time with my buddies at the country club. More time away from that awful house and the woman in it.

Finally, I managed to convince Susan to see a neurologist. Tests. Withdrawal of too many drugs for anxiety. Referrals to psychologists and counselors.

I was not ready to hear the words "Dementia, probably Alzheimer's." Those concepts were not in my repertoire of life's facets. But they showed up anyhow.

Love tests us all the time.

I have always loved Susan and still do. But this situation is not like avoiding the draft in the 1960s. It is not the same as getting control of the awful variables in life. It will require me to make some serious decisions in which Susan will not play a role. Except as my blameless wife who must endure the results of those decisions.

Chapter 14
Introspection

No husband is symbolic of all husbands. We are all different, just as all wives are different. The same thing is true of marriages.

I am neither a psychologist nor a sociologist. But I am somewhat acquainted with those areas of study. We are daily besieged with stories about human relationships in books and magazines, on television and other electronic media.

Many of my retired friends, women and men, watch TV soap operas. In casual conversation they give details about plots, characters, relationships, and even emotional context. Love, hate, intrigue, deviousness, addictions, ulterior motives, neediness, dominance, vulnerability, evil and the so-called wages of sin.

No, I do not watch soap operas. Although some sitcoms and full-length movies, in addition to both nonfiction and fiction books, are close to the same thing. Some of those are cloaked with more sophisticated terms such as history, government, war, economics, prejudice, politics, even religion.

Please do not think of me as a cynic. I believe in the fundamental goodness of human beings as we try to better understand ourselves as highly intelligent creatures. Most of us are people who work hard to overcome bad impulses. We often lose. But then we seek forgiveness and try again. A cycle.

Media produced by people like us are a kind of literary introspection. A study and commentary on the human condition as we struggle to make sense of our lives. Then along comes something like Alzheimer's Syndrome. I did not expect it. Nor did the fictitious characters known as Mike and Don. It did not hit them directly. Instead, it did something much worse.

It hit their wives.

I do not see myself as being like either the fictional Mike or Don. But my wife, if she could, might argue the point. I agree that I have had my moments. Like the fictional Mike, I grew up in the 1950s. I was an offspring of "The Greatest Generation." Postwar Americans were winners. We won the big war. And, while less well-defined, we prevailed in Korea. We had the bomb.

Although the public had mixed feelings about individual members of the military, subliminally at least everyone was proud of its accomplishments. While many courageous and dedicated women served and died, it was men who played the most prominent role. That appealed to me.

At age 17 I enlisted in the army, right after high school. Afterward I went to college and received an ROTC commission in 1961. My assigned branch was armor or tanks. I became a tank platoon leader and later a company commander. We trained hard for a possible conflict with the USSR in Europe. What everyone thought was inevitable because of the Berlin Wall and Cuban Missile Crises, calmed down. More Cold War. More predictions of an unimaginable Armageddon. But no shots were fired. No bombs were dropped on an enemy. Or on us.

The Kennedy assassination and escalating tensions in Southeast Asia. Vietnam. A revisiting of Truman's "containment policy." Keep the communist countries from expanding. A murderous and insidious soap opera writ large.

Our major involvement in Vietnam started in 1965. Because of the terrain and other conditions, army commanders decided to use lighter vehicles and helicopters. Lots of them. Only the Marines sent tanks, pretty much as mobile artillery. By that time, I had been transferred to the Texas National Guard, allowing me to start my teaching career.

Because my obligation to the service was fulfilled, I decided to leave the military in 1966. I had many reasons. Our involvement in Vietnam did not make sense to me. Guard units like mine were being trained to control anti-war demonstrations throughout the country. I hated the idea of confronting our own people on American streets.

Maybe more importantly, I did not like who I was becoming. Military commanders do not ask subordinates to hold hands, meditate deeply, and conduct long discussions about strategy. Sure, good ones seek advice, but the commander makes the ultimate decision and subordinates follow those orders to the letter. Or else.

That persona can burn deeply into someone who realizes he is solely responsible for making life and death decisions. It is hard to shake off that scenario in civilian situations. In my classroom. In my home. I might come across as uncompromising, dictatorial, demanding—almost an addiction.

My wife understood the problem. She was the daughter of a decorated military commander in World War II. Her mother taught her how to cope with the situation. Because I knew it was becoming a problem in me, I worked with my wife to overcome it at home and in my profession.

While not perfect, I like to think I improved greatly over the years. My wife's strong personality and my need to change perspective to overcome economic challenges, brought me back to better ways of behaving. Unlike the fictitious Mike, it did not take being hit in the face with my wife's Alzheimer's to open my eyes. That enlightenment happened decades before.

As for the fictitious Don, my knowledge of that scenario comes mostly from observation of other guys I know. They often think of themselves as masters of the universe, who marry someone equally ambitious and full of hubris. Sooner or later, they are rudely surprised and cannot believe their world is falling in on them.

I did not give the stories about Mike and Don happy endings. In some ways, there is no such thing. But I can, based on my own experiences, change the ongoing storyline in ways that will soften the outcome.

Chapter 15
Intervention

Writers of fiction know a storyline dictates the ending. But an author must be careful to plant clues in the narrative that keep the reader or movie-watcher a little off-guard. Real human beings and their lives have many and varied dimensions. Characters have awakenings or experiences (plots) that make them see something differently. Something that might make them act differently.

That plotline has happened to me dozens of times in real life—events called "a-ha moments." As a guy entering my eighth decade of life, I try to calibrate my outlook with the daily acceptance of *a-ha moments*. In fact, I search for them.

Critics pan stories, novels, or movie scripts that are too predictable. Readers like to be surprised with plot twists, or characters that turn out to be different than they first appear. We like that approach because many of us do not exude a good "first impression."

How many times have you heard someone say, "He (or she) isn't who I thought she was?"

Let's go back to the story I wrote about Mike, the dogmatic know-it-all man married to Karen. Early in their marriage Karen confronted Mike about his overbearing and domineering manner. Severe physical or verbal abuse was not involved. Mike was basically a good guy with bad social skills. He clearly had an unworkable attitude about how good relations are established between husband and wife. He behaved the way he was taught. The way his father's demeanor taught him.

I did not throw in stressors such as alcohol, drugs, poverty, physical abuse, abject laziness or irresponsibility. Mike was presented as a fundamentally good man, who underneath the crustiness was sensitive and loving. He thought he was doing the right thing and tried to live that kind of circumspect life.

Karen saw how he tried. She knew she could depend on him. That he loved her and would take care of her in any situation. But it was a docile compromise. Docility replaced mild volatility. A little more every year. Confrontation would get her nowhere.

Karen knew women in her circle of friends who would give anything to be in her shoes, those married to unstable men who were weak, addicted, abusive, or irresponsible.

No scientific evidence decrees that depression, by itself, can lead to dementia. But what happens to the human brain when hopelessness sets in? Where is the escape valve?

I once heard someone say there is a difference between being *unhappy* and being **not** *happy*.

Unhappy is active and results in relational disruptions such as arguments and fights. Where *happy* offers feelings of euphoria and delight, *not happy* is a kind of neutral state of being and acting. *Not happy* is an emotional void that is pervasive but cannot be easily explained.

Karen was becoming *not happy*, and that state of mind made Mike *not happy* too. That condition is called stasis or, in human terms, excessive passivity. Karen became depressed and withdrawn. She was more compliant when Mike made demands or non-negotiable suggestions. The situation gave Mike no satisfaction at all, but he felt stuck.

Then Karen started the descent into dementia. At the end of the story, Mike called himself a jerk and dreaded the future. With good reason. He finally had his *a-ha moment*. But by that time, it was far too late.

I did not like the ending of the story about Mike and Karen. No story should end with hopelessness as the only result. But that cannot happen unless there is some kind of *intervention*. Something must be injected into the evolving story that changes its trajectory. A plot twist of some kind. A character who does something surprising.

Will that curtail the possibility of Karen contracting Alzheimer's? Medical science would probably say no. The sadness of her diagnosis would not change. But the runup to the discovery of Karen's Alzheimer's might have been different.

The relational environment Alzheimer's invaded might have become better, thereby lowering the level of trauma in Mike. It would not absolve his feelings of guilt and despair, but the intensity might lessen. How?

I have already admitted to a little of Mike in me. It is much better now than decades ago. But I can still be judgmental and somewhat pompous, delivered in the guise of intellectual inquiry. Clearly, this annoys some people. As it should.

That characteristic is intimidating, and I know it. Yet, as with Mike, it is a kind of compulsion. It shows up when I feel cornered. There is nothing like having a wife inflicted with Alzheimer's to make a guy feel cornered. But Alzheimer's does not care. Its manifestations cannot be backed off with an attitude or the power of combative logic. It makes worthless each utterance and every strategy to overcome.

With Mike and Karen, what would *intervention* look and feel like? An imposed meeting of the minds over a bowl of ice cream before the Alzheimer's became acute? Individual or marriage counseling? Psychological therapy? Separation? Dynamic family conversations?

Toward the end of the story Karen has already made the decision to be tolerant and passive. The storyline suggests Mike caused it, although we do not understand the underlying reasons.

Personality strengths or weaknesses can be either innate or imposed by life experiences. Sometimes both.

The confluence of Karen's passivity, depression and dementia is already such that intervention will not help her. At this point, the focus is on Mike. He knows he is stuck in a lifelong compulsion and is increasingly NOT happy about it.

How can anyone intervene to help a guy who believes he compulsively allowed himself to force the woman he loves into depression? Possibly a melancholy that foretold her descent into dementia, whether that is medically true or not.

But Mike could *think* it is true, that he is making the wife he loves die of a broken heart while in the throes of Alzheimer's. He grieves. He regrets. The grief consumes him and eats away at his mental and physical health.

So intervention must concentrate on the black cloud of grief. It is within that context the storyline must pivot.

Chapter 16
Grief

How is grief disrupted? What intervention in a storyline or real life can either eliminate grief or shove it to the side?

Karen is sinking further into Alzheimer's, and Mike's health is declining because of his self-perceived role as an enabler. Although Mike senses he is not directly culpable for Karen's mental regression, he may have enabled Alzheimer's to enter their relationship. He constantly reprimands himself, *If only I had been a better and more caring husband, this would not have happened.*

After C. S. Lewis's wife, Joy, died of cancer, he wrote an insightful book called *Grief Observed*. Lewis listed and commented on the commonly understood stages of grief: shock/denial, anger, depression, bargaining, and acceptance.

Lewis suggests that the stage of shock/denial is closely related to fear. Mike is certainly afraid, and I can relate to that feeling. Fear of the unknown. Fear of being left alone. Fear that my actions precipitated this awful thing in my family. And guilt. Plenty of guilt.

About anger, Lewis says we want to blame someone or something else for this desecration of life. But that piece of the storyline will not work. Mike and Karen were not singled out. Alzheimer's is an epidemic, and Karen became part of it.

Depression is another word for ongoing sadness. A sadness that never lets up because it is based on what might have been. Why can't we just go back to the heady days of our youth? Depression is also an epidemic in our society, for many more reasons than Alzheimer's.

The fourth stage, bargaining, is probably where intervention has the best chance of making an impact. As awful as Alzheimer's is, and as many mistakes Mike made in the years leading up to it, it has been a learning experience. Maybe Mike has learned important lessons about himself and his relationships. Medical science indicates that Karen was probably genetically predisposed to being a victim of Alzheimer's.

The same way some people get diabetes, cancer, and a myriad of other disorders. It just happens. Our job, as those who love the afflicted person, is to stay positive and do all we can to help them through this unwelcomed part of their lives.

With the stage of acceptance, Mike can find ways to move on with his life, having learned difficult and valuable lessons. He can be productive and have positive relationships with others, even while taking care of his wife the best way possible. He can become proactive, learn about support systems in our society and take advantage of them. Make new friends.

Bargaining and acceptance could have been plot twists in the Mike and Karen story. Mike's a-ha moment might have been the introduction of a counselor, therapist, or close friend.

Interactions with other caregivers. Reading helpful literature. A relative with the ability to have an effective heart-to-heart conversation. Those are all possible ways to intervene, to disrupt grief.

Another caregiver who had already gone through those stages of grief. This caregiver convinces Mike there is a light at the end of the tunnel. Maybe a loving daughter or son spent time with Mike and convinced him that their mother is not a victim of Alzheimer's because of his behaviors. All those interventions are possible. Even plausible up to a point.

But my own story is not like Mike's. I, the man who invented fictitious Mike, do not have a good frame of reference. My wife was no shrinking violet in the years prior to the onset of her Alzheimer's. She was her own woman, something I discerned early on. She had substance and conviction. We deeply respected each other. And there was the ice cream pact we agreed to, although occasionally we gave each other a reminder.

Have I gone through the stages of grief? Yes, but they were mitigated in several ways.

One important part of the storyline for Mike and me is that neither of us are misogynistic. On the surface, Mike might come across as believing men are superior to women. But that is untrue. Some men are genuinely misogynistic. I find that attitude despicable.

Mike's problem is a kind of misguided chivalry. He plays a role akin to Lois Lane's Superman. Mike never wanted to demean Karen. He loves her. While his relations with other women are rough around the edges, he is cordial and respectful.

Mike is basically a good fellow who wants to do the right thing. He likes and respects their female friends. Those friends realize he has a domineering attitude within the home, but they can kid him about it. Jokes. Laughter. Evidence that Mike is more vulnerable than he would like to admit.

That candor opens the door to a wide range of possibilities. Open discussions about emotions, help with day-to-day events caused by Karen's decline, conversations about options, speculating about the future and how to plan for it.

Those female friends, with husbands often included, intervene better than anyone else. They help Mike better manage his growing despondency, all-consuming guilt and grief.

How about that for a plot twist? The man who was compelled to manage his wife's life and felt guilty about it when she contracted Alzheimer's, is lifted out of his debilitating grief by other women.

Chapter 17
Insight

Novelists and screen writers love stories about privileged and wealthy people. Men and women who, after years or decades of living what appears to be the good life, are hit with almost unimaginable tragedy and heartache.

Success is rarely linear and achieved in an unimpeded fashion. Challenges along the way create bumps in the road. But they are overcome with grit and determination. Until they are not.

We challenge the elements and prevail. We succeed financially and materially. All is magical until reality hits us in the face with obstacles we cannot overcome. Sometimes those obstacles are of our own making—our hubris and unacknowledged failings.

Perhaps the reason for the success of storylines and screenplays has to do with our need, as ordinary folks, to know ALL of us are only human. The temporal aspects of money, power, privilege, pleasure, and unlimited opportunity will someday end. We cannot predict how everything will finish, but the events leading to the end will likely be multifaceted. Different dimensions. Awful events such as accidents over which we had no control. Illnesses that seeped unexpectedly into our bodies. Cancer. Alzheimer's.

The end of a multifaceted successful life is too often not included in planning by the story's main characters. Youth. Good health. Money. Decades stretch out in front of the couple.

The only choices to make are associated with the right universities, wedding venues, honeymoon trips, new homes, cars, birthing and raising successful children, and how to fill the time with pleasurable pursuits. Family, friends, interesting things to do. And the commercial world of advertising lays out the entire menu everywhere you look, in every kind of media.

The story of Don and Susan, *Success is Multifaceted*, was an opportunity to firmly declare that nothing we do as human beings, no matter how well-educated, wealthy, or privileged, will help us defend against life's gremlins that sometimes morph into monsters.

Even when we live in a social bubble. In big homes on lovely, gated properties served by the best public or private schools. Entertained by country clubs with beautifully manicured golf courses and tennis courts. Alzheimer's does not respect privilege. Nor do many other human afflictions.

My wife was a fan of Eleanor Roosevelt. Not because she was married to Franklin. Not because she was the nation's first lady for many years. Not because she belonged to a certain political party.

Barbara was impressed with Eleanor because they believed in the same things. Eleanor stood up for the defenseless. She was an advocate for the disadvantaged. With all her money and privilege, Eleanor took great risks to support those who were disenfranchised. She held to her convictions and was a substantive human being committed to others.

Eleanor's life was one of service, no matter the sacrifice required. And she did not mind disagreeing with her handicapped husband, the president, if she thought he was wrong. She even stood up to the family's grand matriarch, Sarah Delano Roosevelt, Franklin's mother.

Eleanor was not complacent, nor was she impressed with wealth and social standing. Most historians agree that Franklin would have never become president without Eleanor's dedication and amazing initiative. Neither of them would have gained the White House if they had not demonstrated an altruistic faith in people and a herculean determination to serve.

How does someone become like Eleanor Roosevelt?

What if my story line for Don's wife Susan had given her the personality of Eleanor Roosevelt? Would Don have picked her as his wife? Probably not, given his preference for living a docile luxurious life. What if Susan was interested in international relations because of a deep need to help the world's downtrodden people? Yet Don chose Susan for his wife.

The laws of mutual attraction among human beings are mysterious. Maybe Don saw something in Susan he had not seen in anyone before. A depth of character. A unique way of believing. Something he learned about and wished he possessed.

My wife helped me understand the importance of helping shunned and disenfranchised members of our own society. Susan might have convinced Don that life can be just as much about altruistic service as making a nice salary in the comfortable corporate world.

Perhaps Don and Susan make a pact to serve a world larger than themselves. That idea is not as farfetched as it sounds. Wealthy people occasionally show up in the newsfeed, consumed with a need to serve the underprivileged and underserved throughout the world.

Despite Susan's kindness to mankind, will she still become afflicted with Alzheimer's in my storyline? Yes. Will Don consequently suffer? Yes. Will Susan's dementia-related meltdowns never happen when her mother has the accident and dies, and when her daughter contracts breast cancer? We do not know, but suppositions can be made. Suppositions are never supported by fact.

But as a husband who has spent many years with a wife in the shadows of Alzheimer's, and as a daily visitor to her memory care home, I can tell you what I *sense* is true: women who know they are loved and respected for having made real contributions to the welfare of others seem more content. Even within the fog of Alzheimer's.

Just as feelings of love seem viable and evident in the afflicted brain, so does the knowledge that a life has included meaning and significance. Sometimes it comes out as a radiant smile, a muttered word or two, a quick sparkle in the eyes, or a look of serene satisfaction on the face.

Medical researchers might laugh at my plot twist. Those of us living in the reality of an Alzheimer's diagnosis might not.

We all die. Our hope is that we die with the knowledge that our life meant something, and we were appreciated for it. Although we might manage our storyline differently, Alzheimer's can still become a reflection of life's meaning.

Chapter 18
Bill

My name is Bill, and my wife's name is Patricia. Seeking forgiveness is the most difficult experience of my life. Television in the late 1950s often filled afternoon time slots with old movies. Many were westerns and war movies from the 1930s–'40s. On hot summer days I would stay inside and watch them on my family's seventeen-inch Sylvania Halo Light.

One day I saw a 1941 movie titled *Sergeant York*. It was a biopic of a man named Alvin York, who transitioned from being a conscientious objector to a decorated hero in World War I. Alvin was a young Christian man living in rural Tennessee when he was drafted to serve in the American infantry. He became conflicted about why he was given so many accolades for the killing or capture of German soldiers.

The movie was well done. It was used to help elevate patriotic enthusiasm for our country to get involved in World War II. Until the Pearl Harbor attack, many Americans wanted nothing more to do with foreign wars. Pearl Harbor, along with patriotic movies such as *Sergeant York*, changed everyone's attitude almost overnight.

We are products of both our era and our culture. In the late 1950s I enrolled in the ROTC program at my high school. Only boys participated. And it was popular.

Although the stalemate of the Korean War was discouraging, our nation was clearly leading in the Cold War.

The decade of the 1950s also saw a resurgence of both religious beliefs and dedication to service. I was caught up in both because of church activities and summer camps. It was also a time when programs sponsored by the Boy Scouts and YMCA were a tremendous influence on young men like me from certain segments of society.

Both my future wife, Patricia and I, graduated from high school in 1960. Both of us decided to attend a local vocational/technical school. She was trained in the culinary arts while I learned how to become a diesel mechanic. Patricia's parents owned a restaurant and she planned to work there after graduating from the two-year program.

I was always a good mechanic. And the growth of the American trucking industry seemed like a terrific opportunity for me. The military draft was something young men needed to take into consideration. While in the vocational/technical school I was able to get a deferment, so that allowed me to plan for both a vocation and family life.

Patricia and I were married the summer of 1963. I found good employment and as expected, Patricia worked in her parents' restaurant. In September we learned we were expecting our first child.

We joined a church. We liked its emphasis on strong moral values, allegiance to Christ's teachings, and belief in the salvation Jesus gave us by sacrificing his life and rising from the dead. The congregation was also committed to service of all kinds and members included multiple World War II veterans.

It seemed right for the cross to be directly in front of the sanctuary with the American flag prominently displayed on the right. Belief in God through Jesus Christ and belief in American values. What could be better?

The military draft loomed large in our minds. Everything in the world seemed so unsettled, especially after the Cuban Missile Crisis. And we kept hearing about the little war in Southeast Asia—how our country might become involved in a small nation we had never heard about. Vietnam.

Patricia and I had long talks about our future. I thought my skills as a diesel mechanic would be of great value to the army. But veterans at church said I would be less likely to be given that assignment if I waited to be drafted. It would be better to enlist. So, I did.

Patricia and our newborn daughter were welcome to stay at her parents' home until I could arrange for them to join me in a suitable deployment.

My three-year stint in the army began with basic training in the fall of 1964. After basic training I was given my MOS, military occupational specialty. In the paperwork, I stressed my talent and training as a mechanic.

But I made the mistake of mentioning my skills as a marksman during the high school ROTC days. Like Alvin York of World War I, I was a crack shot with a rifle—with awards to prove it.

Veterans in my church said my skills as a diesel mechanic would be valued stateside or in Germany, because all the new M-60 tanks were diesel. Unfortunately, they were not the officials making job assignments in the regular army. Those people thought I would be better suited as a sniper. I objected to that assignment—to no avail.

About a year later I was sent to Vietnam and assigned to infantry units as a sniper. In today's military such an arbitrary assignment would be seriously reviewed on many levels. However, in 1965, assignments were made where soldiers with special skills were most needed.

My job was to kill individual human beings classified as the enemy. Thoroughly camouflaged and from hidden locations. My assigned objective was to bring down the morale of the enemy, to disrupt its leadership, and to save lives of my fellow Americans who could be killed by enemy soldiers in machine gun nests. From trees. Coming out of tunnels. Dropping mortar shells on our lines. My job was to spread fear and confusion among those enemy soldiers.

Yes, I received medals for my work, and I rose to the rank of staff sergeant. My assignment after a year in Vietnam was as an instructor of novice snipers. And my discharge from the army was honorable.

But thou shall not kill. How could I reconcile the meaning of the cross and the American flag in our church? They stood only a few feet apart. I felt like both a patriot and a sinner.

With treatment for my PTSD, I eventually managed some of that reconciling. And Patricia was always there when I woke up from my nightmares. She told me time after time I was not a sinner and that she loved me.

We prayed together often. She held my hand when I begged God for forgiveness. Without Patricia and our God, I would not have survived those years. She helped me believe God is ever present in our lives.

Now that woman who saved my life in so many ways is fading away. And God seems to be going with her. Did God abandon us by giving her Alzheimer's?

Our children came out okay, for which I am grateful. But they live far away. Patricia has gone to a memory care facility. Now I am alone with my demons. With a pervading feeling God has not forgiven me for my sins.

Chapter 19
Choices

Bill and Patricia are the fictitious couple who graduated from high school together in 1960. They attended trade schools to learn culinary arts and diesel repair. Nice kids. Responsible, moral, and religious people making right choices for their lives. Doing everything as they should. Giving thanks to God for the privilege of living in this country and worshipping as they please.

I struggled to write that story but felt it was necessary. The year 1960 was pivotal in many ways. It was a collision point between faith in God-given possibilities and the emergence of bad choices made by the world's leaders.

That was my era, too. I could not disguise the reasons behind Bill's PTSD. Reasons for his guilt and believing he had sinned. Believing that his sins, the killing of so many people, might have something to do with Patricia's decline.

Was God making Patricia pay for his sins? Why would God take away the one person in the world who could keep him sane—make him feel as if his life was worth living?

My army experiences were divided between service as an enlisted man right after high school graduation and commission as an officer after college graduation. Half and half. Although I was assigned to a combat branch, I was not sent to Vietnam nor did I experience the trauma of a shooting war. Just lucky. The army did not tactically use main battle tanks in Vietnam. It was not that kind of conflict.

Over time I met many guys like Bill. I still do, as an AARP volunteer concerned about the welfare of retired veterans.

Rewriting the storyline for Bill and Patricia was more difficult than other fictitious scenarios for two reasons:

The first reason was Bill's inability to psychologically "compartmentalize." The psychological condition called "cognitive dissonance" means being unable to separate religious beliefs and the sniper assignment Bill was given.

No one is sure why some people can dissociate value systems and others cannot. The military is finally aware of the problem. It is one thing to expect a pilot to press the button to fire a missile or drop a bomb on an unseen enemy. But it is quite another thing to ask a man to aim at a person's head or heart and pull the trigger.

If I had been one of the veterans in Bill's church, those who suggested he enlist rather than wait for the draft, I would have had a serious talk with him about how military decisions are made.

Bill was impressed with Sergeant York's exploits as a military hero in World War I. York did not just object to his assignment in the infantry. He made an issue of it. He had a heart-to-heart conversation with his commanding officers about his Christian beliefs regarding the killing of another human being. They listened. Then he was given time to reflect on his concerns and make his own decision. York chose to fight because he felt the cause was righteous.

But York was not proud of what he had done. He did not believe he deserved all the recognition he received. He just did what his nation asked him to do in the name of righteousness. As far as I know he did not suffer as badly as Bill from PTSD.

The second reason an alternative story line is hard to write is the naiveté on the part of both Bill and Patricia. Their outlook on life was characterized by nearly absolute trust in authority figures, the belief in leaders or systems that seemed indisputable. Excessive obedience to authority.

I am not a professional psychologist, but I know something about that discipline. Both religious belief and patriotism can tend toward absolutism. Charismatic authority figures convince others as to exactly what is right and what is wrong. The history of humankind is rife with such extreme ways of thinking and acting. The results are almost always disastrous.

As educators, my wife and I encouraged our students to think. To analyze. To examine all dimensions of an issue, thereby avoiding simplistic solutions to complex challenges.

My fictional Bill and Patricia were raised with absolutes. Right versus wrong.

❧❦❧

I walked into my battalion's office for the first time as a wet-behind-the-ears Second Lieutenant. Behind the commander's desk was a life-sized picture of General George S. Patton. Hands on hips. Two ivory handled revolvers on each of those hips. Bigger than life—almost godlike. A face filled with resolve, a demeanor exuding confidence in himself and his rigid set of beliefs.

These lines actor George C. Scott recited in the opening of the famous movie were direct quotes from the real Patton. "Now, some of you boys, I know are wondering whether or not you'll chicken-out under fire. Don't worry about it. I can assure you that you will all do your duty. The Nazis are the enemy. Wade into them. Spill their blood. Shoot them in the belly."[2]

My job was to ensure the five tanks I commanded would annihilate the enemy. That was Patton's credo—the absolute to which I was expected to pledge myself.

Did I accept that absolute? Yes, but in the context of doing my job well and fulfilling the oath I took: "I do solemnly swear (or affirm) that I will support and defend the Constitution of the United States against all enemies, foreign and domestic; that I will bear true faith and allegiance to the same; and that I will obey the orders of the President of the United States and the orders of the officers appointed over me, according to regulations and the Uniform Code of Military Justice. So help me God."

An intervention for Bill, either before or after Patricia's diagnosis of Alzheimer's, would need to expose his misunderstandings of the oath he took. He could have, as York did, take advantage of the military justice code. But it was too late for that.

The more significant intervention in the past or the present, would be his view of authority and his interpretation of authoritative pronouncements. Slowly, it might be possible for sensitive veterans, both men and women, to help him understand that all human beings live with contradictions every day.

That does not make them sinful.

It just makes them God's children who seek the right way, while acknowledging and trying to do something *positive* about overcoming their failings.

Chapter 20
Sam

My name is Sam, and my wife's name is Julie. I learned there is no such thing as taking someone for granted. Sometimes that is not understood until it is too late.

I cannot remember a time when I did not know Julie. We were born close to the same time, in the same hospital. We grew up together in the same neighborhood. We attended the same elementary, middle level and high schools. Our families attended the same church.

Some people even thought we were siblings. Blond hair, slender build, same accent, and common interests. Julie was kind of a tomboy. She loved daredevil activities and was always competitive. Until our teens she could run faster and jump higher than any of us guys.

When we were twelve Julie was a good two inches taller than I. Smarter too. Her report cards were always a notch above mine, in almost every subject. Most of the guys did not like Julie. Because of their attitude, I tried to dislike her too. It did not work.

As children we were always able to talk about everything. She seemed to respect me and listened. And I wanted to listen to her. About how dumb our parents were. About teachers neither of us liked.

Eventually the awkward years arrived. As juniors in high school I shot up two inches taller than Julie. My athletic prowess was greater than hers. We noticed we were becoming different people with varied interests, odd impulses, and more sensitivity to the opinions of others. Everything became more complicated.

After high school graduation we decided to attend different colleges. I went to a state university in the southern part of the state and majored in engineering. Julie attended a small private college in the state west of ours and majored in nursing.

In the early 1970s, I received a college deferment from the military draft. By July 1, 1973, it did not matter. Compulsory selective service was over. So was the war in Vietnam.

Julie and I saw each other on school breaks and occasionally during the summer. Nothing much. A lunch or two. Maybe a walk in one of the parks. Although we were young adults, the carryover from our earlier years persisted. We discussed our studies, dates we had, interesting things we were involved with: clubs, sports, trips.

Each of us had been serious about other people, learned difficult lessons, and eventually broken up. It was hard to explain why our personal relationships with others regularly failed. Neither of us were willing to admit that the nature of our long-held friendship might have something to do with it.

After graduation we both found good jobs. I became an engineer in a heavy equipment corporation, and Julie was an emergency room nurse. We worked in cities seventy miles apart, but in the same state.

No internet then, just the phone and post office. So we wrote letters and occasionally talked. Sometimes we scheduled lunch or dinner together in one of our cities.

The pattern of our lives in college persisted into our daily routines as workers. On again, off again relationships. Nothing serious seemed to stick. We each had a few friends but spent lonely time in our apartments.

One day I was in a battle with my new CATIA computer, a device that used software designed to make every engineer more productive. Toward the end of the day I threw up my hands and yelled, "That's it!"

The guy in the neighboring cubicle asked, "What's *it*?"

I mumbled something about my frustration of having to learn an entirely new computer program. But that is not what I was thinking.

That night I called Julie and asked her to marry me. I told her whatever it was we were doing was not working, at least not for me. After she got over the shock, she said she would think about it. Might be better if we did not talk about something like that over the phone. So we made a date for dinner the following weekend.

Our discussion was more like planning a merger. She thought it would be advantageous for both of us, but there was much to consider: Which job would be given up, where would we live, how we would explain it to our families, and what date would be best?

We said we "cared for each other" but the "L" word did not escape our lips. All the details of the merger were mapped out and executed efficiently. We married. The two of us were finally together on a permanent basis, and our lives were better for it. A few years later we had a child together. We enjoyed a happy family life.

Our son Clay was a cheerful little guy. We enjoyed taking trips and doing all the things happy families do. Over the years Clay grew up, spoiled as only children often are, attended college, and entered a secure profession.

Both Julie and I stayed with our professions until we were in our late 60s. We traveled to places in the world we always wanted to visit. Took cruises. Hiked and camped out a little.

Occasionally we were challenged by a little medical scare, but we both stayed in fairly good shape. Our daily routine was familiar and comfortable. Nothing spectacular. A nice arrangement.

Then came the Alzheimer's diagnosis. Julie's occasional forgetfulness was getting chronic and even frightening. The doctor said she was not certain how rapidly the syndrome would advance, as every case was different. With some people, it took years to develop. In Julie's case it was quite rapid. Too quick.

I watched her asleep on the bed, sensing she would be a different woman when she woke up. Subtle maybe, but still different. Every day. Almost every hour.

Could I be in love with this woman? I must be—because this was agony. Why could I not detect my real emotions years ago and tell her how I felt? Would she have been able to reciprocate, given the way our relationship formed?

I guess I will never know.

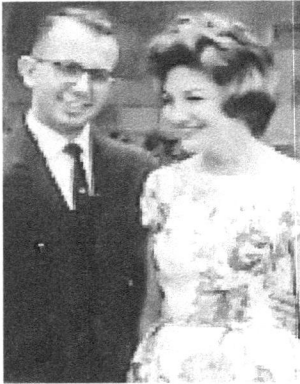

Barbara and Stu April 1962
Fort Hood, Texas (Picture 2)

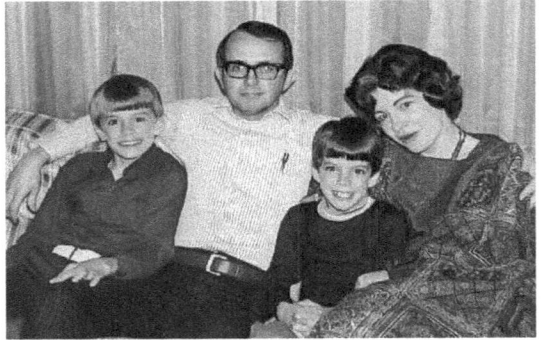

Ervay Family in 1974 (Picture 3)

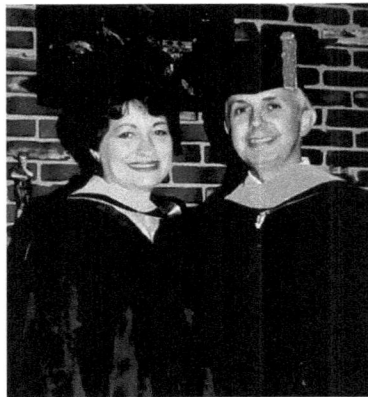

Barbara Receives Master's Degree
in 1987 (Picture 4)

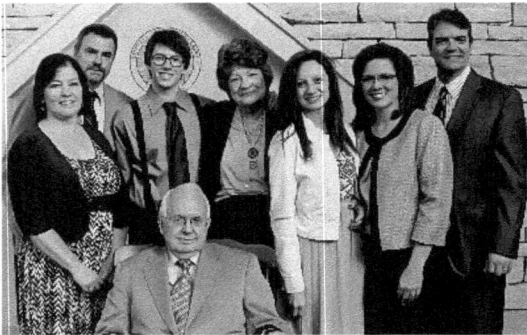

Ervay Family at Stu's Retirement in 2014
(Picture 5)

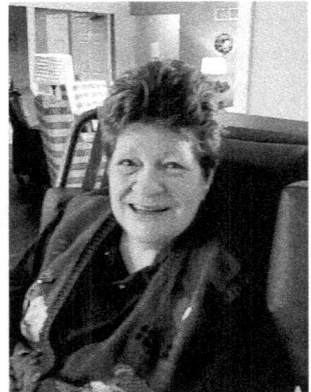

Barbara in 2018
Prairie Elder Care (Picture 6)

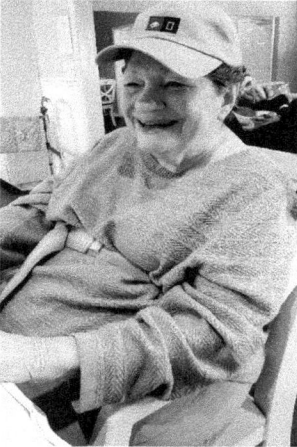

Barbara in 2018
Prairie Elder Care (Picture 7)

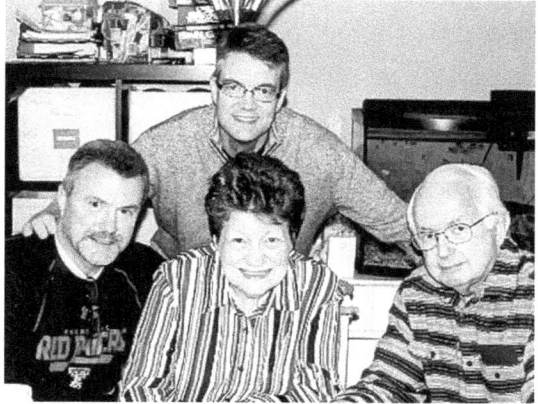

Ervay Family in 2018 at Prairie Elder Care (Picture 8)

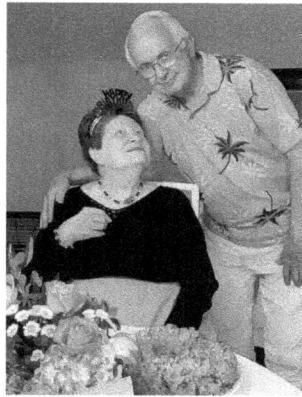

Barbara's 79th Birthday
Prairie Elder Care (Picture 9)

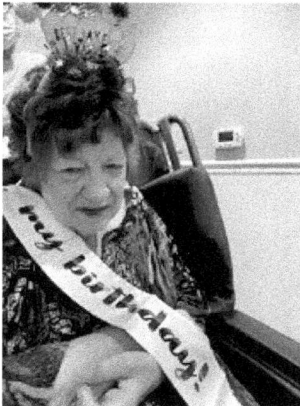

Barbara's 80th Birthday
Prairie Elder Care (Picture 10)

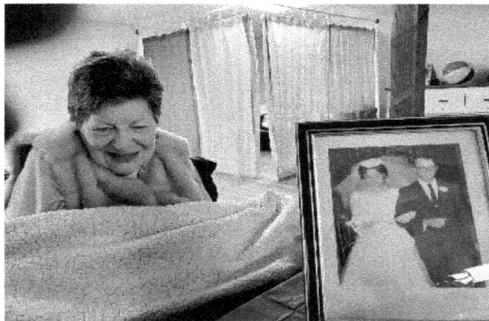

Barbara on Valentine's Day 2020
Prairie Elder Care (Picture 11)

Chapter 21
Practicality

Sam and Julie, the key players in a matrimonial merger, lived together for practical reasons. Their story line may sound odd. A man and woman brought together based on the proximities of time, space, and circumstances. Nothing more.

It may seem strange to us in our modern world, but not within other cultures or time periods in history. Marriage was often seen as an economic or political necessity in which human notions of romantic love had little or nothing to do with it. So practicality in marriage, or even cohabitation, is therefore not an oddity. It has been around for centuries and is even encultur-ated in some regions of the world today.

As an AARP volunteer, I know many older widowed couples will link up with someone either in marriage or as a live-in companion. My mother did, and I thought it was wonderful.

It occurs now for various reasons:
- To relieve loneliness
- To overcome economic challenges
- To mitigate medical caregiving needs
- To eliminate property maintenance issues

But fictitious Sam and Julie were in their late thirties when they decided to merge. Who knows what their day-to-day life was like over the decades they were married. Their relationship while growing up seemed to be perpet-uated in adulthood. Clay's birth tells us the relationship must have included special moments.

The French use the term, *ennui*. It is a kind of boredom that comes from living in an emotional vacuum, an existence in which no one is either happy or unhappy. Just an easy, comfortable, predictable, routine existence punctuated with brief moments of either joy or sadness.

An ennui marriage is just a necessary burden, but one worth enduring because it is safe. Safety is all its participants expect.

The storyline for Sam and Julie is significant because their merger-like marriage lasted decades. They raised a child. They grew old together. The connection they made as children was a strong bond, no matter what they called it. An ongoing acceptance of the status quo, day after day. The problem with that kind of relationship is that it allows complacency. The "other" has always been in "my" life and things will continue that way. But we know this is not true.

In Sam's case it was Julie's Alzheimer's journey that awakened debilitating effects on Sam's emotions. Maybe even his mental health.

Psychologists, therapists, and pastors tell us we should talk with each other before the inevitable arrives. *Really* talk with each other. But more important is the need to talk about how we *feel*. Especially how we will likely feel when the time comes to part—through death, debilitating physical disorders, maybe even Alzheimer's.

My wife and I discussed end-of-life contingencies. We started by writing a will after my brother died at age thirty-one. He left a widow and two daughters. Our first will concentrated on who we wanted to care for our young sons if we both died. Decades later we set up a comprehensive trust. Estate stuff: power of attorney, wills, distribution of property, and other mundane but important considerations.

Those were the practicalities. Talking about our feelings was something else altogether.

We began talking about feelings started when our parents became ill and died. How we missed them! How we felt like orphans after the last parent died.

How strange it felt to be moved to the front of the boat.

One of the most difficult movies for me to watch is *The Remains of the Day*. I keep thinking the butler, Mr. Stevens, will finally wake up and realize what a fool he is. Duty. Precision. Robot-like devotion to duty. A measured and orderly life that ignores all the passions around him and the obvious love Miss Kenton has for him. When he does come to his senses, it is far too late. The Miss Kenton he once knew disappears from his view on the back of a passenger train. Like Julie disappears into the fog of Alzheimer's.

I could have changed the story line for Sam and Julie. The death of their parents or some other dramatic event could have been written in, causing them to change the regular routine long enough to address the future. In *emotional*, not just practical terms. Ways that might cause them to admit they are people with feelings, vulnerabilities, weaknesses.

Like Joy did for "Jack" (C.S. Lewis) in *Shadowlands*. She helped him understand that happiness and pain come to all of us, and we must work through it. Like it or not.

For some reason we men put up emotional barriers to certain kinds of realities, so it takes the unrestrained emotion of women to break down those barriers.

Miss Kenton did not do that with Mr. Stevens. She suffered quietly and let Mr. Stevens go on with his dismal little life. To the end.

Real life is not written by a guy like me who manipulates the storyline any way I wish. We, the participants, write our stories. The best way to do that is for the people involved to open the door and effectively, sensitively grapple with whatever future walks in.

Chapter 22
Ken

My name is Ken, and Darlene is my wife. A new reality is never easy because its conditions seem unfathomable. Especially when we are not ready.

Isn't it interesting how often the word "institution" is avoided by the medical community? I do not blame them. All I can think of when I hear that word is a large building or facility in which many people live or work in accordance with specific rules and behavioral expectations.

Another image that comes to mind about institutions is overbearing efficiency, orderly ways to work with large groups of human beings. For men my age, the example that comes to mind is the military.

How impressed I was with basic training and army operations in general. The management of barracks, food service, clothing and equipment, cleaning and maintenance, training schedules, medical and safety precautions, and coordinating our transition from civilian life to becoming soldiers.

While military institutions are efficient and tailor-made for training large numbers of people to participate in war, they are also dehumanizing. Recruits were prepared to become cogs in a machine that would effectively fight similar machines sponsored by the enemy.

Reflecting on those early days in the military, I remember feeling scared, disoriented, homesick, and resentful. I resented losing my independence—my sense of individuality. My security as a member of a loving family and community. I eventually got over it, but it was not easy.

The army knew I would get over it. In fact, many people learn to accept military life as a new kind of family, a new security with different ways of thinking about community. But an ultimate acceptance of a new way of life leaves those left behind with feelings that range from proud to a sense of abandonment.

My wife Darlene knew about the military. Her father was in the Marines during World War II. He was killed on Okinawa. Her mother remarried, but Darlene and her sister were treated too sternly by their stepfather. He was never physically abusive, but more of a demanding martinet than a loving presence.

The time I spent as a draftee in the army was something I coped with, but never adopted as a way of life. I was every bit a "citizen" soldier, having done my duty as expected then moved on with my life.

During the year and a half we dated, Darlene and I talked about her complicated life. My own family was warm and loving, so we aspired to creating a loving family like the one in which I grew up. And we did it. Two boys and a girl. Healthy, few problems in school, and a happy life together.

In her 60s, Darlene's mother, Betty, was diagnosed with Alzheimer's. As her dementia worsened, the stepfather vacated his spousal responsibilities and initiated a divorce. His abandonment left Darlene as the primary caregiver. Her sister lived in another state.

I did all I could to help, which involved financial assistance when Betty finally had to be checked into a care facility. An "institution" in every sense of the word. The authorized facility was large, dramatically understaffed, and smelly. Betty sat in a wheelchair all day. She was poorly groomed, essentially ignored by individual staff members responsible for nearly twenty additional residents.

The entire experience was awful. No money was available to cover residential costs. Eventually we had to seek Medicaid coverage.

Doctors told Darlene, "There's a good chance you'll someday be afflicted with Alzheimer's. Heredity, you know."

They were right. A few years later in life than when it attacked her mother. Given everything she endured taking care of Betty, Darlene was petrified about what might happen to her.

I was her only lifeline. Her only "champion."

Darlene apologized repeatedly for what I was facing. With our financial situation, we had few options in terms of hiring outside assistance. For hours we talked about how to keep Darlene at home. Could we find friends and other relatives to help? Receive assistance from our sons and daughter without burdening them too much?

It was exhausting. I tried to stay strong for Darlene. Read everything I could on caregiving at home. Over time I found a few answers. Hints in books, literature produced by organizations such as the Alzheimer's Association, ideas from friends who faced similar challenges. I even located a few of Darlene's friends who had available time. They were willing to give me a break occasionally when the situation required it.

But then it came time to put elevated security locks on the outside doors. Do the best I could in the kitchen. Install a chair lift because Darlene's back pain increased going up and down stairs. Clean. Make the bed. Play old DVD movies she enjoyed. Then play them again. Many times, over and over. I never paid much attention to Darlene's side of the closet, her cosmetics or lingerie drawers.

But I learned. The friends who offered help took care of her hair, and I drove her to the salon when we could afford it. Then she forgot how to use the shower and flush the toilet.

With each Alzheimer's stage she entered, I felt pangs of anxiety compounded by oppressive claustrophobia. My world was closing in. With each breath I felt less on top of the situation. A friend finally said, "It's time."

I knew she was right. My wife could no longer stay in the home she loved. I had to break my commitment to her. At this stage of her cognitive functioning she would not, could not understand.

With the help of one of our friends, I found a memory care home, one of the many I had already checked out. It had a vacancy. Smaller and better staffed than others, but it smelled clean. Nevertheless, it was still an "institution" with schedules, rules, supervision, tidiness.

So I made the necessary arrangements, signed the contract, and drove my wife to a place she never wanted to go. A place I never wanted her to go. It was the hardest thing I have ever done, and I felt as abandoned as she did. She did not, could not understand.

Why was I doing this to her? All she wanted to do was be with me in our home.

Chapter 23
Promises

Ken made a promise to Darlene, these two fictitious people who had reason to fear institutionalization. Both subconsciously knew it was a contingent kind of pledge. Only a *hope* that Darlene would be kept at home through the caregiving years. The attempt to somehow control the future was important to both of them.

Predictably, when Alzheimer's is involved, the promise of keeping the afflicted loved one at home is often broken. But Darlene's plea that she be kept at home until the end was understandable. Especially given her childhood experiences.

Those experiences started with losing her father in the war. Then she acquired a cruel stepfather who abandoned her mother, Betty. The stepfather walked out the instant Betty showed signs of dementia. When that happened, Darlene's fears were amplified by having to assume caregiving responsibilities for her mother. Then having to help her mother resort to the use of Medicaid and a substandard long-term care institution.

I wrote the fictitious story about Betty's situation with gloomy underpinnings. Darlene realized a similar future could await her. The fictional scenario might have been much worse, based on daily reports we hear about the deficient care of elderly people. Abuse, accidents, understaffing, incompetence, as well as deaths from viruses and other preventable diseases.

Darlene's fear put an enormous amount of pressure on her husband, Ken. The emotional response I wrote into his story was also mine. Panic attacks and severe feelings of claustrophobia.

For me, those reactions were in addition to bouts of depression which are more common. Unlike many men, my reactions did not result in some form of medical emergency.

At the end of the scenario, I did not discuss Ken and Darlene's finances. Betty qualified for Medicaid because she was living below the federal poverty level. She may have also qualified for a myriad of other reasons.

The bottom line underscores that Betty was destitute and could prove it. Ken, Darlene, and other members of the family did not have the financial resources to help.

To use an archaic term, Betty essentially became a "ward of the state." That term is no longer a legally correct designation, but it is similar to what happens today. Governmental funds took care of Betty.

How could Ken and Darlene pay for Betty's care in a residential care facility? Darlene was concerned about their limited resources. Financial resources are a big deal on many levels.

Ken found an acceptable memory care facility where he could enroll Darlene as a full-time resident. How he planned to pay for her care was not mentioned in the story I created. I gave Darlene a sister, but she could not earlier assist with their mother's care. Were things different now? Possibly Ken's parents both died and gave him a nice inheritance. Or not.

And how about their three adult children? Maybe one or two of them were prospering in a fine profession and had a bundle of cash. Perhaps one of them married rich. Maybe one of these prosperous adult kids was loving and generous, pledging to do anything to ensure good care for their mother.

A fiscal fairy tale might come true. It happens all the time. Even if such a circumstance happened, Ken would still suffer from breaking his promises to Darlene. He would feel all the associated guilt. But at least he would not need to worry about money issues.

What would happen if, instead of a fiscal fairy tale coming true, Ken was looking at a possible financial disaster? Less than $150,000 in savings with a monthly salary of less than $5000. No long-term care insurance, a remaining house mortgage of $125,000 with a monthly outlay of over $2500. Mortgage payments, insurance, utilities, home and car maintenance, food, pharmacy, small incidentals. And even more bills if there is any kind of health emergency of his own.

Ken is now sixty-seven, so he can collect the second-tier amount in Social Security and qualify for Medicare. Darlene would also receive something from Social Security and be qualified for Medicare. Those things help.

But Medicare does not pay for residential or even in-home care. Except when a patient qualifies for Hospice services. While helpful, Hospice assists with quality-of-life problems in patients not expected to survive the disability. Darlene has not reached that point.

Residential care costs are not covered by Medicare, so Ken is looking at shelling out over $5800 a month for Darlene's basic care. If he continues working, stays healthy himself, and Darlene lives many more years, their savings account will be quickly depleted.

It could be worse.

If Ken loses his job due to age discrimination, chronic illness, or disability, he too will need to think about Medicaid as the only remaining option. The rules surrounding Medicaid are complex. Many attorneys specialize in both estate planning and how to qualify for Medicaid. They could help Ken through the maze of options left open to him. But they are not cheap, even when fees are partially covered.

How should I have written the story line of Ken and Darlene? In some ways it does not matter. There is no happy ending in terms of how guilty Ken feels about breaking his promise to Darlene. He will likely be depressed over time. But, as with me, his emotions might become less intense. At least about Darlene.

What happens to him otherwise, in the context of his own health and management of finances, might be a different story.

Chapter 24
Bud

My name is Bud, and Billie is my wife. We have been married thirty-four years.

Fifty-four would be a better number, but that will never happen.

Billie was eighteen and I was twenty when we married. Probably too young, but age is just a number. We thought we were mature enough and our parents approved. In a word, we were happy.

Billie supported us through my years in college. Later she completed a secretarial degree in a community college. It worked out precisely as planned. Billie works as a secretary to an attorney. It has been a good job and she has done well.

Our first daughter was born before we could afford a baby, but we made do. Then another daughter, and finally a son, somewhat more planned. Our lives were not perfect, but eventually we could afford a good house in a pleasant neighborhood. The schools were good, and our kids made better than average grades. Both daughters went to college a few years then dropped out to marry. Our son finished college and is now in graduate school, studying to be a nurse.

A few days ago, Billie's boss called me about her behavior. She was making uncharacteristic mistakes at work. "Is she doing that at home?"

"Yes. But nothing significant. A little forgetfulness. Trouble finding the right utensils in the kitchen. Things like that."

Her boss understood but requested a medical opinion. "Multiple mistakes made in a lawyer's office are unacceptable."

Billie and I visited our general practitioner who referred us to a neurologist. Tests were conducted. They eliminated treatable conditions associated with hormonal disorders, infection, or the aftereffects of a mild stroke.

It was early onset dementia which further tests indicated was probably Alzheimer's. No way to know for certain, but it could be "rapid" onset which meant its symptoms would quickly worsen.

Like Julianne Moore's character in *Still Alice*, a 2014 movie. The real person depicted by Moore was fifty-one and died within five years. Basketball coach Pat Summit was diagnosed at fifty-nine. She also died within five years.

For Billie, at age fifty-three, that meant she would never reach sixty. We did not have much time to adjust. To think things through. To talk things out.

But plans must be made. Her job. My job. Finances. Travel modifications. Eventual in-home care. Possible future institutionalization. Long-term care insurance.

It started with periods of denial for both of us, and the eventual crying while we held each other tight. We sobbed our way through the trauma as we faced the loss of a future. The ultimate loss of the magical bond that started over thirty-five years ago.

My friend Jake is a word guy. He does crossword puzzles all the time. We are friends because of our mutual interest in sports—not because of words.

As an engineer, I think words are necessary labeling tools. But I am more interested in numbers. Numbers are exact. Precise. In my profession there is no room for nuances. Subtle differences either are or are not. Words leave too much room for interpretation. However, words are better descriptors of human behavior than numbers, because we human beings are so complex and different.

As Jake would say, our personalities have "shadings" even "contradictions." Those cannot be described in numerical terms. Jake thinks nothing can be pinned down scientifically. An example is that scientists are now backing away from traditional tests of intelligence. IQ numbers are still valid as one indicator of human potential, but not seen as comprehensive as they once were.

Jake was an English major and has been married twice. He is now single and teaches at a local community college. We have known each other since our junior year in high school. As different as we are, two things support our friendship. Sports and his love of our family. All of us. Billie and the three kids. In fact, the kids call him Uncle Jake, and he seems to like it.

His two divorces are evidence of a chaotic personal life, but Jake is philosophical about it. Occasionally he cites some author of classical literature. Stuff that is hundreds of years old. Most of the time he comes across as being a little crazy to me, but he seems to enjoy my puzzled looks.

Jake was as devastated as we were upon hearing of Billie's diagnosis. He was uncharacteristically silent, and a tear ran down his cheek. Afterward the two of us went out on my home's patio.

We just sat there. Then Jake said, "One of my favorite classical authors is a man named George Gordon Byron. Today he is usually known as Lord Byron."

Jerked out of my silence, I said, "I've never heard of the guy. Probably not an engineer or mathematician."

Jake nodded. "He was an English poet who lived in the late eighteenth and early nineteenth centuries. He died at age thirty-six. But Lord Byron led a very eventful life. While writing some of the most significant literature in history, he also pursued other passions. Many of his activities were questionable, and his rashness led to his demise. He died from an illness contracted after a Greek war."

In a poem about war, Byron used the words "fickleness of fate" and "transience of human life." But, according to Jake, those terms can be applied to life in general.

Life is not an accumulation of numbers, of years. Not just two numbers with a dash in between.

How we spend the precious years we are given is more important than the final numerical tally. What Billie and I have done with our thirty-five years together is more important than the number itself. What we do with the next five years is equally important.

Jake asked, "How will you and Billie respond to this challenge?"

"I have no idea, but I guess Billie and I need to discuss it. Soon."

Chapter 25
Numbers

For Bud and Billie, time will slip away. Unrelenting, like watching sand in an hourglass descend from top to bottom. Theirs is a story I hated to write. Not just because of early onset Alzheimer's, but because of how others have suffered from cancer.

In our fifty-eight years together, my wife and I have known and worked with people diagnosed with terminal cancer. Often people much younger than the two of us: colleagues, secretaries, associates. And we have known others who survived probable death by letting their doctors take aggressive measures: mastectomies, hysterectomies, other painful and life-changing procedures.

But those we knew who were not so decisive or lucky were women in their forties with young families. Loving husbands and beautiful children. Outstanding in every way. Sometimes these women were gone within a year.

My wife and I avoided cancer. But not everything else.

In her sixties and early seventies, my wife struggled through many medical problems: a serious potassium deficiency, a painful gallbladder attack, seizures caused by epilepsy, and incapacitating back pain. She also underwent hip surgery and was treated for other breaks after falling unexpectedly. Some benign cysts on her back were easy to remove surgically. But no cancer.

The onset of her Alzheimer's was hard to pin down. Her problems with forgetfulness and other manifestations of dementia were slight in the beginning. Just "senior moments."

Our internist, while suspecting dementia through office memory tests, was astounded that she still enjoyed solving Sudoku puzzles. So he was certain it was not early-onset Alzheimer's.

An early cancer diagnosis is awful. But so is early (rapid) onset Alzheimer's. There are two significant differences:

Cancer diagnoses can sometimes be averted through new and evolving forms of treatment. Unless an inoperable brain tumor is involved, it does not usually shut down cognition.

Early-Onset Alzheimer's cannot be treated definitively. Death will likely occur when predicted and cognition will noticeably diminish each day.

Billie will decline rapidly and die in roughly five years from early-onset Alzheimer's. Each day she will likely feel her cognition diminish. If there is any good news, it lies in the fact that the syndrome will not drag on for a decade or more, exacerbating the suffering of both Billie and Bud year after year. And long-term care will not be as expensive.

※

I suppose there is a reason many men are called "control freaks." It is almost stereotypical that men try to "fix" things that concern them. There is no "fix" to Billie's condition.

However, one reason I wrote Bud's friend Jake into the scenario is because his take on life varies from routine and measurable elements such as medication and rest. And counting the years going by. For Jake, life has nothing to do with numbers. It has everything to do with experiences, reaching out, absorbing thrills, and feeling deeply. He is more fascinated with hedonism and stimulating the senses.

The only way Jake's attitude can be described as service to others is in its uplifting enthusiasm. His exuberance is catching. About sports teams he follows, films he has seen or books he has read, interesting people he meets and places he has seen. Art, music, the soft loveliness of the day.

In some ways Jake wears people out. They often question his morality, but he is not evil in any discernable way. He certainly does not leave a trail of debts, duplicitousness, or tears. In some ways he is just a Peter Pan, the little boy who never wants to grow up. Jake offers a fanciful way to help Billie and Bud—with a serious purpose.

Billie's condition can be managed up to a point, using more traditional techniques. People from the church stop by and tell her how much she is loved, how she is in their prayers. Neighbors bring interesting food, beautifully prepared and tasty. Bud hosts little parties at the house, surrounded by friends and relatives he and Billie love. It is all good. Bud and Billie appreciate the love and concern everyone shows them.

But Jake is almost like *psilocybin*, a drug being tested to overcome anxiety in people with terminal diseases. It is similar to LSD in its abilities to reduce dependencies, depression, and fear. It somehow interrupts the brain's compulsion and fear centers in ways that comfort a patient who knows death is near.

I'm not advocating psychedelic drugs for Billie, nor have I created Jake as a proponent of psilocybin. The purpose is that *both* Billie and Bud need an outside influence. One that creates hope and perpetuates a positive connection between them for the upcoming five years. Jake is the catalyst for that hope and positive outlook.

Fear of death is wired into our psyches because, like loneliness, it is a survival mechanism. Being part of the herd protects us from the tiger. Fearing pain and death protects us from doing something to jeopardize our lives or well-being.

My own problems with severe claustrophobia and panic attacks, while taking care of my wife at home, could be alleviated by a significant distraction. An intense conversation. An eye-opening experience. Marveling at something I had never seen or heard before. Mild sedatives could also help, but a powerful distraction worked better. Something unusual, fun, even dramatic.

That is why I created a "Jake" for Bud and Billie. Somebody like Steve Martin's "wild and crazy guy." The oddball who takes them to the zoo on a whim, or packs them off to see one of his girl friends who is a standup comic in a local club, or who pays for and accompanies them on a weekend junket to Las Vegas.

The Jake I created is more than a "bucket list" guide. He is the exclamation point at the end of the sentence. He is the medium who, through outlandish actions, tells Bud and Billie how much he cares, and relishes the time he spends with them.

Billie may not remember those fun times, but the underlying joy she feels might be perpetuated to the end. And Bud will be grateful.

Chapter 26
Phil

My name is Phil, and my wife is Ann. Life has given me challenges to overcome. I have needed both help and a helpmate. But now the person who has been my loving helpmate needs *my* help.

One night in Vietnam I lay on a muddy embankment. Rain soaked me to the skin and insects gnawed on my arms and legs. The soldier next to me said, "Old men start wars, but young men die in them."

A smart college guy. A philosophy major. But if he was so smart, what was he doing in this mess?

The next day, just as we were moving over the embankment to attack the enemy position, he took a bullet between the eyes. Another young man died in an old man's war, lost in an instant.

A few months later, my body took a couple of hits. One superficial, the other just enough to get me on a plane back to the States. My young man's war was over. In a VA hospital, I recuperated from a leg wound with guys who had more severe wounds than mine. Finally, I was able to return to my parents' home. On crutches, a few days after my twentieth birthday. I thought I was lucky. So did my parents.

Once my wound healed completely, I could take the GRE and get a high school diploma. The piece of paper I thought was useless when I dropped out of school. With a GRE certificate I could go to trade school or get a job that trained me to do something more than fire an M-16. Eventually I passed and tried taking courses in a local vocational/technical school. But I was unable to get into the classroom thing.

About that time my parents divorced, leaving my older sister and me to find our own way in life. My sister married her boyfriend and moved to another state. I never saw her again.

An old high school buddy and I found an apartment and low-paying hourly jobs. In the evenings we bar-hopped, associating with other guys like us. Each day was like every other day. We worked as laborers on construction jobs and built residential homes. The type of homes we would never be able to afford ourselves.

Our existence was aimless and purposeless. I did not tell my buddy how bad my nights were, but he seemed to know. Maybe he heard me walking around my bedroom or watching TV at three in the morning to avoid sleep. To avoid the gremlins and monsters in my brain. Attempting to quiet the emotions that refused to calm down.

Both of us had girlfriends, so it was a come-and-go kind of life, at least as much as we could afford. Alcohol, drugs, and other forms of loose living defined us.

Inevitably, my girlfriend became pregnant. Her family was as dysfunctional as mine. So the only family we had were our social friends with whom we lived and partied. Neither my girlfriend nor I were interested in marriage, but we decided to go through a civil ceremony.

Between her restaurant job and my construction work we had enough money to live, but medical costs associated with the baby's birth caused us to seek charitable assistance. We needed help for housing, food and just about everything else. For the baby's sake, we tried to stop our addictions, but that was a losing battle.

Our marriage ended in divorce after the birth of our second child. My continuing problems with addictions, suicidal tendencies, and anger often resulted in abusive behavior. Both my ex and I were deemed unfit parents, so our kids were adopted out.

It was a pattern: another marriage. Another child. Another dissolution of anything resembling a family relationship. I ended up living in a little apartment, trying to exist on occasional odd jobs in the construction field.

Somehow things started turning around. The VA helped and medical treatments for my depression and other issues. A church organization, and a young woman named Ann who was a volunteer. Hazy memories.

Ann was quiet and self-disciplined in a nonjudgmental way. She had a calming voice and manner. Her touch seemed magical with its ability to make me feel at peace with myself and the world. And she was willing to marry the disgusting mess I had become.

Little by little, and with Ann's loving persistence, we started building a real life. It took a while. I struggled with anger, depression, finances, treatment issues, battles with the VA, and other problems.

But we eventually found regular jobs. With my newfound stability, I moved into a supervisory role in a construction company. We lived in a small but pleasant home with good neighbors. No more kids. We became members of a nearby church.

PTSD was still part of my life, but it no longer totally controlled me. Ann's voice and good common sense somehow blocked out the demons in my brain. Life made more sense to me. Together, Ann and I were able to give it real purpose. Our purpose.

One day Ann told me some members of her family contracted Alzheimer's or some other form of dementia as they aged. There was a chance she too would be afflicted.

"We need to talk about it," she said. So we did. For hours. Planning was essential, including getting me, a guy who had needed help all the time, to the point I could be a caregiver myself.

We studied and attended seminars. I concluded that the first few years of ordinary Alzheimer's care was something I could handle myself—*if* I could keep PTSD at bay. *If* we could manage our finances adequately and prepare for the social and medical services to care for both Ann and me.

We had no long-term care insurance. Even if we qualified, the premiums were more than we could pay. We talked with an estate planner, an attorney specializing in our kind of situation. She offered good ideas.

However, unless our financial picture changed dramatically, our only option would be Medicaid assistance. My three children were estranged from me. Neither Ann nor I had anyone else with resources to offer.

An overriding point became increasingly clear. Eventually, little by little, Ann would leave my life cognitively and physically.

That realization was even worse than PTSD.

Chapter 27
Planning

In so many ways Ann saved Phil's life. Could their planning for a future in which she was afflicted with Alzheimer's extend that deliverance from his torment?

Memory is a powerful thing. Especially if it involves a special experience, set of experiences, or significant remarks from a loved one. The loved one does not necessarily need to be a spouse.

My father's observations motivated me to choose a wife with substance and conviction. While my wife's comments were often memorable, it was her devotion to a set of ideals that stays with me, both cognitively and emotionally.

Those ideals do not motivate me to extremes in serving others. But there is no way to escape the need to offer service. Even when tempted to do so. My contributions to AARP, church, education, and others are just a few examples. Even writing this book is something I felt compelled to do.

It is the opposite side of PTSD. A memory that nurtures life. Not one that tries to destroy it.

PTSD is not limited to military experiences. It can come from being abused, denigrated by society for being "different," the victim of a bad accident, or the holder of unusual beliefs.

As I wrote Phil's story, the wartime experience seemed the biggest culprit. But much of Phil's life contributed to his dysfunction. Why did he drop out of high school? Why did he feel a need to join the Marines? Was his parents' divorce based on chaotic relations in the home? Why did his sister move away and the two of them never see each other again? Phil was a fragile guy from the get-go. Horrific experiences in Vietnam cemented his emotional instability and psychological distress.

Although my life was nothing like Phil's, I led many men in the army who were like him. And worse. Much worse. In my years of service, the military gave only incidental attention to guys like Phil. Our job as leaders was to ensure our men were mentally and physically able to fulfill any mission we were given. Nothing more.

I've heard the situation is different in today's military. I hope so.

Ann's character is similar to many women I have known. Strong, resilient, understanding, loving, intelligent and resourceful. Most of all, they are empathetic and selfless. Where do such women come from? I do not know.

Phil was lucky to find Ann. Some might call it serendipity. Others say it was a spiritual gift. The big question is whether the amazing relationship that ensued was strong enough to replace all the bad memories Phil held in his brain. To carry him forward despite future challenges he and Ann were sure to face. What mattered most was that Ann awakened Phil to the way life could and should be lived.

The 2004 movie, *The Notebook*, was based on a book of the same name by Nicholas Sparks. While considered by many to be a great tale, I find the movie difficult to watch.

The same is true when I view one of my wife's favorite films, *Somewhere in Time*. Both are tender and heart-wrenching. The endings are like the one in *Wuthering Heights*, the famous book by Emily Brontë.

Like *Romeo and Juliet* and other tragedies in the romance genre, these stories end with the despair and death of two people in love. My preferred storyline needs to be more inspirational in the context of an ongoing hope and service on earth by the one who remains.

As the author of Phil and Ann's story, I should probably find a way to interject a positive spin. I do not have PTSD or a history of addiction and dysfunction. My cognitive ability and physical health seem okay. Financial security gives me physical comfort. As the one who remains, I am inspired to carry on in ways "we" did as a couple. But I am aware of how fortunate I am.

A recent study by AARP and the National Alliance for Caregiving found that 31 percent of American caregivers consider suicide.[3] Add that statistic to pandemic-charged reports of social disruption and Phil's PTSD would be given plenty of fuel to erupt. The final spark would be Ann's inability to remember Phil or their previous life together.

I titled this chapter "Planning." Superficially, we use that word to describe the act of looking into the future. We try to predict what might happen and how we can be ready when it occurs.

Today most of us view this process in terms of tangibles:

- Money
- Housing
- Food
- Healthcare
- Insurance
- Activities
- Investments
- Communities
- Support

All those tangibles are important. They needed to be discussed by Ann and Phil, which led them to a specialist in estate planning—an important move.

But Ann had an even bigger challenge. In addition to coming to grips with her own decline, she had to emotionally, maybe even spiritually, prepare Phil. She did not hold the romantic view that Phil's life should end with hers, either in the context of Alzheimer's or physical death. To Ann, Phil's experiences and contributions after her departure needed to be meaningful until his own natural death.

Perhaps Ann was able to convince Phil on her own through long conversations or maybe with a trip, such as Joy suggested to C.S. Lewis in *Shadowlands*. Maybe with the help of a pastor or a professional therapist. One who would still be in Phil's life after Ann passed.

Perhaps a notebook full of little letters, or video clips of their conversations, or the continuing of a hobby they started together. Anything that might draw Phil into a world they once shared and enjoyed. A place of emotional space in which communication was perpetuated.

Stories are just manufactured realities. Authors can end them any way they wish. But sometimes they work in real life. We can only hope the one Ann and Phil uses meets their shared goals.

Chapter 28
Frank

My name is Frank, and Jean is my wife. We worry about money and a possible future without enough of it.

Jean and I are nearing retirement. Neither of us is in good physical health, and we both have family members who died of dementia. Probably Alzheimer's. I am already seeing evidence that Jean may be heading in that direction: confusion, forgetfulness, frustration. And she is only a year older than I.

I work as a technician in a local HVAC company, and Jean is physically disabled. We have decent medical coverage and a good 401(k) plan, plus other savings I accrued from a previous job. That total is now about $275,000. Jean served for years as a church secretary. She has no benefit package, but she does receive about $1200 a month from Social Security.

One daughter still lives with us. She is employed full time by the city library and makes $13.50 an hour. One of our sons is in the navy. The other is a graduate student in biology and receives a stipend as a research assistant. Neither is a financial burden for us.

However, we can never look to our children or other members of the family to financially assist us. Our daughter might be able to help in the home, but she plans to become independent like our sons.

Our parents are deceased. We inherited small amounts from them and were careful to invest those assets. Currently that accumulation is about $175,000. Our house is mortgage-free but old, requiring considerable maintenance. Taxes and utility bills are about average. Both our cars are paid for but must be insured and re-licensed every year.

Jean and I would like to travel and are trying to figure out how to do that when I retire. But some types of travel are expensive, so we are not letting ourselves get excited about it.

I will not be eligible for mid-range Social Security until I turn sixty-seven. My employer might keep me on the job two years after the standard retirement age, but much depends on my health and how responsible I will need to be for Jean's care. Although my eligibility for Social Security begins at sixty-seven, we will receive Medicare when I turn sixty-five in two years. Jean will also receive payments, in addition to what is already available because of her disability.

At about $500,000, our inheritance and my 401(k) accumulations seem healthy. Eventually, Social Security will pay us both a total of $3800 monthly. Jean will continue to receive $1200 a month for her disability.

The monthly gross income from Social Security will come to $5000, an annual income of about $60,000. Our other assets are the $500,000, the value of the house, and the two cars. In the current market the house is worth about $200,000, and I have a full life insurance policy with a death benefit of $50,000.

We talked with an estate planner. She thought we were in good shape as we contemplated retirement. We would be covered by Medicare Parts A and B and able to buy a supplemental insurance policy for a reasonable monthly premium.

The estate planner believed we could use some of our savings for travel without risking too much. Standard medical needs could be easily taken care of. Drugs, doctor visits, hospitalization, rehabilitation if needed. Even Hospice services would be mostly covered by Medicare and our supplemental insurance.

There was only one unknown. Caregiving for one or both of us should we contract Alzheimer's. A fiscal swamp since Medicare does not cover extended professional in-home or full-time residential care.

Intermittent care, yes. But *not* full-time care. Either extended in-home or full-time residential care is costly. For example, if Jean's Alzheimer's progresses so quickly I cannot take care of her at home with or without help, we could be looking at an extra monthly outgo of $5,500 for residential care. And that was the cheapest I could find.

Jean might share a room with someone else in a facility that has a resident-to-staff ratio of twenty to one. A top-rated facility would cost as much as $8000 a month or more. Annually that comes to an outgo of between $66,000 and $96,000.

Alzheimer's is different for every patient: behavior patterns, how fast the individual deteriorates, when the person requires additional staff help for managing everyday activities. Many challenges from one diagnosis.

Contracts usually provide for increases due to inflation and additional fees if more staff services are required. In brief, with so many variables, it is difficult to predict costs.

What if I budget an annual amount of $75,000 for covering costs in a moderately good facility, but Jean hangs on for four years? The cost calculates to a total outgo of about $300,000—assuming I do not also contract Alzheimer's.

While the half million dollars we have in reserve once seemed enormous, it could melt away in a few years. In the worst-case scenario, Jean might need care for over five years. Our children would need to find a way to cover costs for my care.

In a short time, we could descend financially from a responsible middle-class couple to dependency on federal and state resources. Our state has not approved something called "Medicaid Expansion." The rules for using government support are both stringent and limited.

Our daughter and estate planner are examining all options. Together we have approached the local chapter of the Alzheimer's Association, the state's AARP unit, and a new program sponsored by the National Association of Area Agencies on Aging: *Dementia Friendly America.*

It is comforting to know some organizations are interested as we walk through the decision-making minefield. But even they cannot assure we will enjoy the "golden" years worry free.

Chapter 29
Money

Frank and Jean are not poor people, but they have discovered a vulnerability—a major threat to their finances. The proverbial *good news and bad news* of human life. The good and bad news scenarios overlap based on a health-related continuum. Medicare, the *good news*, supports that continuum for most physical illnesses.

If a disability does not involve a reduction in cognitive functioning, the afflicted person can mentally participate in caregiving processes. That often allows in-home care, supplemented with incidental outside assistance.

The *bad news* is Alzheimer's. Medicare and other forms of insurance do not support full-time assisted living which is a necessary service as the syndrome advances.

I live in a +50 community in which many couples take care of each other. It works well if both partners communicate cogently. If both stay mentally and emotionally healthy enough to keep the relationship moving forward. Some may struggle financially, but Medicare and other forms of insurance keep them afloat. The continuum may fluctuate, but it remains good news in terms of money.

That is *not* true when dementia enters the picture. The continuum tends to drift from bad news to worse news. In terms of money, physical decline, and emotional stress. There is no Medicare safe harbor. If the situation degrades further, the couple or the family ends up in a financial salvage yard called Medicaid.

The tug of war called American politics sabotages solutions to problems such as those encountered by Frank and Jean. In a different political reality, Medicare might be expanded to include *some* coverage for long-term assisted living. That day may come, but not soon.

Alzheimer's and other forms of dementia have already reached epidemic levels in older Americans. It is expected to become much worse as people live longer and costs increase.

Unless a cure or better forms of treatment are found, memory issues and other disorders could almost bankrupt our country.

In the meantime, Frank and Jean are doing everything they know to do. I purposely created Frank and Jean as responsible and hard-working Americans. They pay their own way in life. They save money. No one in the family is addicted to drugs, alcohol, gambling, or anything else. Their lifestyle is not extravagant. The house and cars are paid for. They do not take expensive vacations. They exercise and eat right.

Yet they face the possibility of financial difficulties if Jean's Alzheimer's worsens. At some point, Frank might hope that Jean's long-term care is shorter than expected. He would hate himself for thinking that way because he does not want Jean to die. But years of expensive custodial care seem like such a waste.

Hundreds of thousands of dollars to care for a human being, albeit his wife, to live in a near vegetative state at $6500 a month. What if he ends up the same way? Surviving only because Medicaid pays for his demented survival in a subpar facility. Bad news morphs into worse news.

The only way to put a more positive spin on the story of Frank and Jean is if they purchased long-term care insurance while in their forties when premiums were comparatively low. Coverage was good then, with a payout of over $100 a day for five years for each of them. That would cut their custodial costs nearly in half for five years of coverage.

But I eliminated that element of the story because, like many couples, Jean and Frank did not think they would need long-term care. Today, finding long-term care insurance is a challenge often prohibitively expensive.

Given that both Jean and Frank are now over sixty with pre-existing conditions, they would not likely find available policies. If they did, the annual premiums could be $5000 or more with possible increases at the discretion of the company.

On the plus side, long-term care costs in the Midwest are less than costs on the east or west coasts. Sometimes much less.

Notice I included *networking* in the storyline. Frank and Jean are working with an estate planner, always a good move. With their daughter's assistance, they are also reaching out to organizations focused on challenges such as theirs.

What Frank and Jean did in terms of networking is unusual. It is amazing how many people would rather avoid making connections during retirement. Some do. They gather for breakfast at McDonalds or participate in a diversion: playing card games, watching soap operas, engrossed with sports either as a participant or spectator, and working with hobbies. Others stay active with various church functions.

There is nothing wrong with diversions and socialization. But the kind of networking I am talking about is more focused on making contributions, doing more than just coping. Learning about options, available support systems, and other community-based structures that keep everyone connected.

One of the first actions I took as an Alzheimer's caregiver was to reach out to AARP. I made an intentional effort to meet and become friends with my neighbors, joined a small and supportive church, and continued professional affiliations as much as possible. And I made sure my family was always in the loop one way or another. Staying engaged was imperative for me.

However, the kind of critical engagement I am thinking about is with service organizations. Those connected with governmental decision-making bodies and community-based support systems. Organizations that actively study problems older people face. Groups that are sensitive to all challenges associated with Alzheimer's and are either willing to do something about them or locate people who can.

One of my professional colleagues was fond of saying, "Always keep stirring the pot. You never know what might pop up!" He was right.

Chapter 30
Contingencies

Using big words is my weakness. I am not trying to impress people with these words, but they express *exactly* what I mean. No beating around the bush trying to explain something in a paragraph when one word does the job. *Contingency* is one of those words, a concrete descriptor of *what will happen given certain conditions*.

A contingency is neutral and depends on understood and explainable circumstances. It is an educated guess based on certain facts. To the extent we human beings plan for the future, contingencies can be written as "what ifs."

People my age lived with "what ifs" all the time. What if a nuclear bomb dropped on us? A planned contingency was a fallout shelter. What if I was drafted to fight in Vietnam? A planned contingency was to flee to Canada, rebel by burning my draft card or give in to the system and do my best to serve.

A contingency is making decisions based on what we know about the realities of life. And it can be *cause and effect*. If this happens and I take a certain action, this effect has a good chance of being the result.

Life can deliver unexpected blows. It happens to people all the time. Most of us do not live a serendipitous life like Forrest Gump. Some good things happened to him because innate characteristics turned lemons into lemonade.

The scenarios I added in this book are different from mine. Situations vary. In some ways I am fortunate. Alzheimer's did not enter our married life for about fifty years. Other significant health issues did not appear during that time. Our relationship stayed intact. We have supportive families. I stayed well and have the resources to take good care of my wife.

But many people are not as fortunate. Their stories are often layered with tragedy on top of tragedy.

I did not want to emphasize that kind of misfortune too much, but just enough to acknowledge that my experiences are *not* standard. In many ways they are not typical at all. Just one man's story that might be helpful to others.

One universal aspect is that Alzheimer's differs from other end-of-life tragedies. The two worst aspects of the syndrome in America are *the effects it has on caregivers and finances*. A large percentage of caregivers report serious problems with health and depression. And finances can take a big hit, even for a family that has planned well.

Other problems may occur prior to a full Alzheimer's diagnosis: depression, memory loss, bizarre behaviors, suicidal tendencies, anger, and unpredictable actions. These are manifestations of suffering, but they can often be controlled with drugs or different kinds of care. On the plus side, Alzheimer's does not typically involve excruciating pain and incapacitating, physical problems which are commonly seen in cancer and other debilitating diseases.

Should a young person or a middle-aged person develop "what ifs" for Alzheimer's? Maybe, depending on the family history. But how about cancer and other afflictions, accidents, abusive behaviors, suicide of a loved one, divorce, financial reversals, and a multitude of other situations that unexpectedly happen?

For a person to do contingency planning for everything would be exhausting and depressing. And it might be a waste of time given all the possible "what ifs." Is contingency planning something that can be painted with a broader brush? Like a way of thinking and being?

For example, I have never thought of myself as a victim. Probably something to do with my loving upbringing and admonitions from my parents telling me I can do and become anything if I want it badly enough.

My family was lower middle class, partly because of the Depression of the 1930s and World War II. My mother's health was also a factor, prompting a move in late 1945 from cold and wet New York to dry and sunny Arizona. My mother refused to be a fatality, a victim to the harsh northern winters. She did not want to die in her forties as her mother did. She refused to be a victim, and my father was the same way.

But later in life my father was afflicted with mild dementia. Not Alzheimer's, but the result of hypoxia, lack of oxygen to the brain due to a mini stroke. With the help of the family, my mother took charge. She refused to let that situation make either of them victims.

The "I will not be a victim" mindset will not overcome all the challenges in life. History is full of horror stories like the Holocaust—strong people overwhelmed by circumstances over which they have no control. But for most of us, the "I will not be a victim" mindset forces us to discover ways to control our own destiny, at least to some degree.

Essentially, there are three parts to the "control your destiny" outlook. The first is *taking control of self-perceptions and actions*. The second is understanding how our world works. The third is *devising and using strategies for meeting its challenges*.

And contingencies? They are important aspects of parts two and three. Knowing what the contingencies are and figuring out a way to deal with them.

Chapter 31
Happiness

One thing I enjoyed about my wife was how she could be unbelievably optimistic, sometimes like Pollyanna.

Pollyanna was a character in popular children's books written by Eleanor Porter between 1913 and 1915. Classics my wife read as a little girl in the 1940s. In Porter's stories, no matter how awful things were, or could be, Pollyanna happily saw the good side. Almost annoyingly so. As a little boy those books were not on my reading list. My view of life has been realistically positive.

When I look at my wife now, hunched over in a wheelchair, I can see her smile. When I ask, "Are you happy?" she will often whisper one word, "Definitely." Something in her brain tells her she is not a victim, even within the fog of Alzheimer's. Somehow, she is in control of her destiny and knows it. In her cognitive and spiritual existence, she understands her world as it is now. And her strategy for meeting that challenge is to see the good side—to be Pollyannaish.

I am happy she can be that way. And I envy her.

As the caregiver of a wife with Alzheimer's, I am neither Pollyannaish nor do I feel like a victim. The life I have today was always something I expected as a possibility in the repertoire of challenges. Planned contingencies were needed.

Those challenges could not be described or pictured in exacting detail. They were just *variations on a theme*. The theme loomed large with frightening components. Alzheimer's or another kind of dementia was one of the components. One of many *variations*.

As a volunteer leader in AARP Kansas, I have immersed myself in studies associated with caregiving.

Recently I expanded my range of interests within AARP. Now I seek ways to meet a challenge issued by Jo Ann Jenkins, the organization's CEO.

In her book, *Disrupt Aging: A Bold New Path to Living Your Best Life at Every Age*, Jenkins lays out a multipart plan. As shown in the book's title, she strives to help all of us think and act differently about growing older. No matter what age we are now.

After reading Jenkins' book, something new dawned on me. Why does American secondary and post-secondary education *rarely* cover all the essential aspects of adult life, including what it takes to be happy?

Schools prepare adolescent and young adult students to be responsible and productive citizens. Students in upper grade levels are prepared for a vocation or profession. In brief, they are taught how to pursue the American ideals of life and liberty.

Life in terms of showing students how to live comfortably and work productively. *Liberty* by ensuring that students understand the rights and responsibilities of citizenship in a democracy.

But where in schools are students taught the basics of happiness? Assuming happiness is an outlook that makes living worthwhile at every stage of life.

What makes people *happy* can range from the highest, most moral of aspirations, to the basest impulses of humankind. The ways people *pursue* their ideal of happiness also extends from enlightened to vile.

But I believe there is a happiness middle ground, related to how we manage our day-to-day lives, year after year.

One chapter in Jenkins' book is titled "A New Vision for Living and Aging in America." In that chapter she describes four freedoms. *Happiness* is one of them. Others are the freedom to *choose, earn,* and *learn.*

Those three "freedoms," unlike happiness, can be achieved if we carefully examine options, make informed decisions, create possible contingencies in case of roadblocks, and stay true to our course of action. Informed choices, strategies to maximize earnings, and the self-discipline to constantly learn. We have the freedom to become involved in those three ways of behaving.

But our society and education do not always help people take advantage of these freedoms. Too many people make bad choices, discount the importance of financial independence, and scoff at opportunities to learn.

Persons oblivious to those three ways of behaving can suffer later in life. The same is true if they are unable to take advantage of these behaviors for some reason. They become a burden to themselves and to the society in which they live. American culture reveres self-determination and achievement as an individual strength. There is much to be said for that belief.

But we as a society are quick to overlook the horrific impact of a poor education system: a dysfunctional family, the challenges of disparity, the lurking catastrophe that lies behind disease, accidents, economic downturns, and a myriad of other unexpected influences on life.

How can we plan for being happy with the knowledge the world may fall in on us any minute? How can a husband plan for being happy when he knows his wife is likely to contract Alzheimer's? Or is now dying from it?

Happiness will not be achieved by pretending, like Pollyanna, or wishing for it. Paraphrasing Jenkins, we need to find a *path to living our best life at every age*.

And we need to manage our destiny by controlling our self-perceptions and actions. By understanding how our world works. By devising and using strategies for meeting its necessary challenges.

"Happy" partially emerges when goals are met. It fully emerges when the "I" becomes a supportive "we." Together, contingencies are identified and dealt with. Then victimhood is squashed.

Chapter 32
We

At this writing, the world is still in the grips of COVID–19. Meanwhile the United States is experiencing a long overdue social revolution. Many of us are living apart from other people: those in our families, workplaces, and churches. We are unable to join others in restaurants, entertainment or sports venues. While I, a husband of a wife with Alzheimer's, am limited to visiting her just thirty minutes a week—outdoors and six feet apart or by using Facetime technology.

Nonetheless, I am acutely aware of how fortunate I am. Living comfortably in a spacious retirement villa in a somewhat pastoral suburban community. Enjoying social time with neighbors in the evening. Having access to social media. Being able to connect virtually with other people and engaging involvements.

And I am grateful for my comparatively good health, the ability to use my brain to take care of myself and engage in one of my favorite pastimes: writing. I am just as grateful for the connections I have with the wonderful people in my profession as we deliberate ways to help schools and colleges during this strange time.

I also celebrate associations with new friends in AARP and the developing relationships I found in the writing community. Those folks teach and guide me into new ways of thinking—even new ways of being. By listening and responding to the feedback they offer, I feel more engaged with life.

Attachment to a powerful "we" makes getting up in the morning worthwhile. Unlike thousands of other people, my existence is not limited to the suffocating "I." So far, it is still a "we" world for me.

And that makes a major difference as I work through my years as a caregiver to a wife with Alzheimer's.

The life I lead today was not a precise contingency I planned in my twenties, or even in my sixties. But it was in the ballpark, given what I learned about the vicissitudes of life. The unpredictability, surprises, and mysteries that make the year-after-year existence on earth interesting.

But remember the pledge I made to never become a victim—a pledge that was not Pollyannaish? It was realistic, given the nature of human existence. To control self-perceptions and actions, seek an understanding of how the world works, and create strategies for meeting challenges. Those three goals were baseline elements of a pledge, although it was a pledge taken mostly from naivete.

Looking back, I inadvertently took advantage of three of the four freedoms Jenkins talks about in her 2016 book. To *choose*, *earn*, and *learn*.

Like many young adults, choosing was difficult. As a high school senior, I considered journalism, law, and the military. I became a journalism major in a community college and joined the army reserve. Two sidebar experiences during those first two years of college shifted my goals. The first was a developing interest in leading young people, primarily in the church I attended. The second was a growing awareness within my army reserve unit that I was a good instructor.

So I became a church youth group director and instructor in the army reserve with the rank of PFC. My self-perception shifted. Without an educated or professional mentor, I began to better understand how the world worked.

The first perceptual shift told me I enjoyed being around young people, so would do better as a teacher than a writer. The second perceptual shift told me that army PFCs do not typically lead and teach. Officers do.

So I created a strategy for becoming both a teacher and an army officer. I "earned" a teaching degree and an army commission. As I went through those preparation processes, I *learned to enjoy learning*.

Previously, like many young boys, I thought school was a necessary stage in life, just something to be endured as a boring rite of passage. Somehow, I was fortunate to mature into a perspective on life that was purposeful. Exercising the freedom to choose, earn and learn.

But I do not remember being happy during that time. Jenkins says we can choose to be happy, and I did. But "choosing" was a far cry from meeting that goal. *Satisfied for the moment* more accurately described my feelings when I graduated from the university and again reported for army active duty, this time as an officer. And I wondered what I got myself into by being assigned to an armored division during a particularly tense period in the Cold War. Mostly I was nervous about not measuring up. But I did.

The realization I could do what was expected of me in challenging circumstances made me happy. Happy to earn the respect of those I worked with and led. I became firmly aware of happiness being a "we" thing.

Companionship alone was not the "we" milieu I needed. In the 1960s it was being part of a band of brothers who faced tremendous challenges. It was the knowledge I belonged to the team and could hold my own in the face of danger. My friends could depend on me, and I could depend on them.

Happiness for men and women. The knowledge we are connected to others with like aspirations. Belief systems with an especially important caveat, a critical extra consideration.

That refers to the quality of actions that make us happy. Happiness can be the offshoot of evil as much as good. Human beings can be collectively caught up in horrible movements, such as the Nazis in Germany, the criminal mob in countries around the world, and other movements that follow a charismatic leader. Understanding that human penchant, we can also explore mentorship or its broader application: education.

As Jenkins said, "We have the right to be happy." We can choose to be happy. I have chosen to be as happy as possible while serving as a caregiver for a wife with Alzheimer's. But that happiness is not to be achieved at her expense, shunted away, or forgotten while I pursue other diversions.

At some point in my life I was mentored, or educated, to be a different kind of man.

Chapter 33
Mentoring

Having a good mentor while growing up is necessary. One who mentors by being a role model as well as a teacher. Benefitting from that kind of mentoring model is in many ways better than a formal education or participating in an apprenticeship, because it can imprint our personality.

Mentoring goes beyond mere thinking. It influences our way of living and being. Sometimes it becomes inherent to a culture. Certain ways of being have been imbued in some cultures so much they become stereotypical: politeness, a strong work ethic, being clean in mind and body, and open to others.

That kind of personality-molding takes time and is sometimes inconsistent. Role models are human, so they can make mistakes in the mentoring process. But they work at staying consistent so those looking to them for guidance are not dispirited.

From a young age we are inclined to be like the adults we admire, often our parents. But not in every dimension of learning and becoming. As we move through adolescence, we often question adult mentoring. Questioning authority is our way of asserting independence, of learning how our talents and interests align with the society into which we are slowly becoming members.

We continue to seek role models we admire, and we want those role models to mentor us in some way. The mentors we select, and what they choose to emulate, is of critical importance to the society we enter when adults.

In the how-to-live-a-responsible-life category, my wife and I had good role models in our parents. Worthy mentors we loved for guiding us in good directions. Marriage. Raising children. Living within our means. Working together for the benefit of the family, both immediate and extended. Our parents taught us how to *pursue happiness* in the context of living responsibly every day. Their guidance, and our acceptance of it, turned out well.

But is living responsibly the sole purpose of our lives? According to Jenkins in *Disrupt Aging*, it is not. She cites Thomas Jefferson's definition: "The best life includes contributing to the well-being of others."

In other words, we should be mentored to live responsibly ourselves *and* help other people. The mentored one must in turn mentor others. The modern term for that behavior is "pay it forward," a phrase created by Lily Hardy Hammond in her 1916 book, *In the Garden of Delight.*

To my wife and me the practices of living responsibly and paying it forward were intertwined. One practice was not possible without the other. Responsible living was the foundation for serving the other, for mentoring or paying it forward.

Hypocrisy, or talking one way while behaving another, has unfortunately become too common in American society. Mentoring is worthless when the person providing the service, or "paying it forward," performs conversely— the mentor is a poor role model. Purposeful ways of living, no matter how well intentioned, can collapse when there is a disconnect between lifestyles and mentoring efforts.

All of us are susceptible to hypocrisy. Mentors and the mentored, no matter what status in life, can experience the lines of communication being irreparably severed. The problem is that mentors can overreach. Some do it intentionally for personal aggrandizement. Making money.

Getting elected. Becoming popular. Being loved. Others do it for altruistic reasons but make a mistake.

Was I mentored to be a husband responsible for taking care of a wife with Alzheimer's? No, at least not in the specifics. But I was taught how to avoid being a victim. The mentoring I received included the recognition of contingencies, and I was taught how to be resourceful.

Jenkins' term for being resourceful is to always ask ourselves, "What's next?" Then we define and seek the good life.

The job of answering the question, "What's next" was something my wife and I did together. Goals emerged from that discussion. Strategies were developed, and the whole thing was done within our vision of what the good life should be.

That is no longer part of her destiny. But it continues to be part of mine.

The knack of being resourceful on my own has diminished. I do okay but dread the day I get "the call." That my wife has died or entered the end-of-life scenario for Alzheimer's patients. No longer eating because she cannot swallow. It is inevitable. And it will change my life.

The caregiving responsibility has covered many years, and I hope I have done a good job. I know what to do when the phone call comes. All those contingencies are planned and paid for. Our sons know what to do. So does our church and others who support us.

But I have come to dislike the word "widower." How does a man married fifty-sight years plan for that? Where is my mentor, my role-model? How does a widower have a good life?

Associated with the search for mentoring is my need to find where I belong. I am a retiree who, according to popular priorities, belongs with groups who enjoy their golden years in places where everything is done for them. Smelling the roses. Singing old favorites. Enjoying casual conversation. Playing golf.

When the time comes, my job will be to figure things out. Writing this book is meant to be an exercise in mentoring and belonging. Writing something I hope to continue. I will do the best I can to continue being a role model for men, and perhaps women, of all ages.

Chapter 34
Belonging

Sociology was a challenging field of study, but it frustrated me. I did not understand it, because the subject was too subjective. How does one research a topic with so many variables? Human beings are too unpredictable and hard to classify, especially when it comes to their behaviors, their needs and beliefs.

Researchers prefer patterns, systems, cultural rules. Such as, "Given these circumstances human beings are likely to behave like _____."

In American society, whatever is written in the blank has a good chance of being wrong. The ties that bind us together are unraveling exponentially. This cultural change has given our nation multidimensional characteristics, especially when it comes to belonging. Historically, this situation in our young and diverse nation is not unusual.

The question can be answered more accurately when studying smaller, isolated tribal groups, especially those in which survival depends on a unity of belief and action. In smaller tribes of human beings many behaviors are so enculturated they are not only predictable but expected. Examples include the Amish and other small, sectarian groups in the United States and around the world.

However, most Americans cringe at living such a life. Freedom is our mantra. Freedom is our Constitutional right. Don't tread on me. "Belonging" to some folks is a synonym for captivity. Commitments are either avoided or given a contractual exit option. Allegiance is conditional.

I am struggling with the disparity between needing freedom and a sense of belonging. The pandemic has exacerbated that struggle everywhere, including my little segment of society.

Months ago, since my wife was stable and well taken care of, I decided to take a trip on my own. A place both of us had on our list of preferred destinations but did not have a chance to take: Costa Rica and the Panama Canal. It was a National Geographic trip on a small vessel. Regular communication with home was spotty with only expensive email and a ship-to-shore phone for emergency use.

The trip was all I expected it would be. Enjoyable learning experiences, meeting interesting people among the passengers and crew. I missed my wife, but I liked the feeling of freedom as I hiked through rain forests, saw different plants and animals, and enjoyed the canal.

But I felt something else, a feeling I have had on other occasions, a sense of belonging. Like I was part of a wonderful expedition, traveling with people who shared my enthusiasm for the natural world.

Neither my wife nor I felt that way on most other cruises, on floating cities with thousands of passengers. The National Geographic cruise gave me a feeling of intellectual and even academic intimacy. Perhaps because I, and the other passengers were taking the trip for reasons other than entertainment, eating and socialization. It made me feel like I belonged to something bigger than myself in the context of meaning and growth.

It reminded me of an expedition in which I participated as a fifteen-year-old, 168 miles of the Colorado River through the rugged canyons of Utah and Arizona. Dangerous and exhilarating. I felt unbounded freedom, mixed with a sense of connectedness to my friends and the environment.

It became a rite of passage for me—a kind of purposeful freedom. And it was so physically and mentally engaging I remember thinking, "I belong here."

Over the years I have had similar experiences: the military, serving on teaching faculties, participating with my sons in the Scouting program, working with my wife and colleagues in a publishing/consulting organization, staying active with state and national professional organizations.

But now, other than occasional service opportunities, I do not regularly experience that feeling of belonging. With some developing exceptions, I feel neither free nor part of something. Some of the problem is the pandemic, still raging. But the problem existed before COVID–19.

This disconnect is possibly associated with the image linked to aging and retirement. Hundreds of advertisements hit us each day touting the wonders of living in a particular retirement community. The good life for seniors who deserve nothing but the best. The claim is freedom, to do what we want to do and decide when we do it. We belong because we are sitting around a dining table toasting the good life with each other.

What is wrong with that? Retirement homes give us freedom to do what we wish and a sense of belonging in the context of companionship. Speaking for myself, I neither want nor need that kind of freedom or way of belonging.

What helps me now is much more dynamic. I gain freedom by seeking interesting opportunities and reaching out for them. Writing books and other manuscripts. Searching for and finding opportunities to serve. Probing my own creative abilities to determine more of what I can contribute to the world before I leave it.

Success in any of those activities tells me I have the *right to belong*. Not to just take up space with others in my community. I am still a worthy member of this world, nation, society, and my own family.

I can feel my wife telling me, in approving tones, that she is proud of me for staying the course. For continuing what the two of us started.

Chapter 35
Resourcefulness

The word "resourceful" has traditionally meant staying on top of whatever we encounter. Being aware and flexible enough to handle anything thrown in our direction. Responding with a practical, down-to-earth method for meeting challenges or opportunities.

Avoiding being a victim of circumstances. Establishing a mindset that is more proactive than reactive. Utilizing tons of common sense.

Additional definitions include *ingenious, creative, sharp, gifted, capable*, and *spirited*. Or *enthusiastic, ambitious*, and *vigorous*.

These thesaurus-related definitions conflict with my pragmatic, down-to-earth beliefs. They enshrine exceptionality. People who are better than most with the rest of us somewhere in the ordinary middle or below average.

I am a strong believer in science and the scientific method. But I have long believed the variances in human potential defy narrow, mathematically driven scientific classifications. Such as IQ or scores derived from how well students perform on pencil and paper tests.

We have been told the Scholastic Aptitude Test (SAT), American College Test (ACT), and other standardized pencil and paper tests are good predictors of student success. These tests were once in the context of how college courses were traditionally taught, and students evaluated. But today we know they are deficient in measuring *resourcefulness*. When using my definition as being basic common sense and amazing ingenuity.

Public schools, colleges and universities are starting to wake up. Education theorists have now moved *creativity* to the top of preferred learning objectives. Creativity encapsulates *both* common sense and ingenuity—resourcefulness.

My ability to be imaginative in the face of stark realities has allowed me to meet many challenges, conduct problem-solving exercises, and make both practical and unusual decisions. Resourcefulness has also allowed me to seek out and be responsive to recommendations received from others.

It has given me the power to analyze information systematically. It has helped me draw logical conclusions and act on them, then follow up. Above all, my resourcefulness has overcome emotional paralysis.

Many men do not think they can be affected by emotional paralysis. I was one of them. Growing up, my heroes were the resolute and decisive guys depicted in movies and on television. Steely-eyed, righteous, wise, courageous, and strong enough to face almost impossible odds. Leaders among men. Chivalrous to women. Tender with children.

I still get a lump in my throat when reading *Don Quixote of La Mancha*, a book by Spanish author Miguel de Cervantes. The book was published in the early 1600s and is the basis of a 1965 musical titled *Man of La Mancha*.

An ordinary old guy goes cuckoo and believes he is a knight errant destined to fulfill a quest to bring righteousness to the world. He and his faithful servant Sancho Panza ride around the countryside looking for opportunities to serve his quest. Sancho Panza knows his master is a looney old fool but remains loyal because of friendship and recognition of his uplifting motives.

In the musical, Don Quixote sings *The Impossible Dream*, composed by Mitch Leigh, with lyrics by Joe Darion (© 1965).

What hits me every time I hear that song is how impactful it can be to many men who believed and tried to make a difference in the world. Not because they were crazy, but because they needed something inspirational when confronted with an incomprehensible reality.

Like Alzheimer's attacking their wives.

Don Quixote saw giants who needed to be subdued for humanity's sake, when in fact they were windmills. A confrontation with one of them resulted in his being caught in a blade and slammed to the ground. Yet he remained resolute. He used what was left of his addled common sense and ingenuity to continue his quest. Until he encountered The Knight of the Mirrors who showed Don Quixote that he was a mad old fool, convincing him that he was just a dysfunctional and ordinary man.

Ordinary men no longer have a quest for what is best in life. They let emotional paralysis make them lose their resourcefulness. They lose their ability to use common sense and ingenuity to face something like Alzheimer's.

That becomes the issue for men who are caregivers. How many times does the windmill have to slam a guy to the ground? How many mirrors does it take to show him his inadequacies in caring for his wife? The essential question is: How can husbands remain resourceful when the reality of Alzheimer's causes emotional vulnerability, the precursor to emotional paralysis?

How did I become resourceful when others find it difficult? How have I continued to be resourceful in spite of Alzheimer's attack on my wife? The answers did not come in the form of great philosophical revelations or any sort of spiritual awakening.

The answers came mainly from hackneyed phrases I heard while a teenager and young adult. Common clichés used by school friends and military buddies, street corner admonishments I took to heart:

- Don't sweat the small stuff.
- This too shall pass.
- Eat the elephant one bite at a time.
- Use your imagination, stupid!
- Get right back on the horse after it throws you.

I use the word "resourcefulness" as a combination of common sense and ingenuity. Though clichés grow tiresome, they are firmly rooted in earthbound truths. They can be the trigger for setting off an explosion of ingenuity.

By not letting the small stuff bother me, I focus on creating a better solution to more significant problems. By chipping away at solving problems a little at a time, time itself can be part of the solution.

Resourcefulness does not depend on how well-educated we are. It does not depend on being remarkable in some way. All it requires is that we look around and locate strategies that make common sense, then use our God-given and very human ingenuity to act in ways that serve our own needs as well as those of others—especially a wife afflicted with Alzheimer's.

Chapter 36
Purpose

Before our marriage, my future wife introduced me to her family. Her father, a college graduate in architectural engineering, was vice president of a steel fabricating company. Her mother was actively involved in the community. The brother was five years younger and still in high school. Nice family.

They were culturally somewhat different than mine, but compatible enough. My wife's father served as an officer in World War II, so my status as a junior army officer gave us common ground. We were both college graduates. But our purposes for attending college could not have been more different. His purpose was to create products used in building large structures. My purpose was to educate children and young people. The same purpose as my future wife.

On a second visit to the family my future father-in-law gave me a book to read. I do not remember the title or the author, but it was about famous business moguls in America. He did not say why he gave me the book, but the intention was clear. *Those who can, do; those who can't teach*, which is a paraphrase from a George Bernard Shaw quote in his drama series *Man and Superman*.

I was familiar with the term, although in 1962, it did not apply to women. Teaching was believed to be a good profession for females. Like nursing, secretarial work, and similar occupations.

That derogatory quote applied to men. Because *able* men worked in the world of commerce, construction, or industry. Or in professions with real social status such as medicine or law.

Vocations or professions in which the purpose was to contribute to the economy or social structure. To earn a good salary to support a family.

At the same time, I was also being pressured by superior officers to consider a regular army commission. The pressure was not on me alone. During a Fort Hood social occasion, my commanding officer attempted to persuade my fiancé to encourage me to stay in the army.

And my fiancé's father had a serious chat with her about my career choice of education. She stood her ground on my behalf.

We had talked about and agreed on what the purpose of our lives together would be. Purpose trumped other considerations. Living a life of service through education was our choice.

After serving in the military, my plan was to teach high school social studies and journalism, then to eventually become a school administrator.

Finding one's purpose in life is dependent on many factors. It is the most important of all the decisions we make and based on *influences*:

- the family into which we are born
- the culture into which we are raised
- our aptitude, or what we are good at doing
- what we learn to value while growing up

These influences apply to the subject of purpose at any point in life's continuum—not just childhood, adolescence, young adulthood, middle age, or old age.

Purpose is not something issued to us at birth by a domineering society, such as ancient Sparta, where life's purpose for both boys and girls was dictated by the state at an early age. Unlike the Spartans, we can find and choose our own purpose based on faith, introspection, and influences. And tweak it over time.

Our foundational sense of purpose within a free society can be molded to fit different occasions, different problems and opportunities. But it cannot be completely transformed or dramatically reshaped. *Purpose* is not just an attachment to our personality. It is fundamental to who and what we are.

Purpose in caring for a loved one is related to who we have always been and wanted to be. Molded a little differently perhaps, but still an extension of what we cherish, of what constitutes our baseline purpose for living.

The family into which we are born is the first influence on the purpose we choose. Nuclear, extended and adopted. From infancy we watch, listen, emulate, and reflect on how the people around us talk and act. We notice what they believe. How they take care of us. How and what they teach us both directly and indirectly. How we as offspring fit into the purposes of the adults who care for us.

My parents were children of farmers, growing up through two world wars, a horrific flu pandemic, and a devastating economic depression. Their purposes evolved from survival, which meant knowing how to stay ahead of pending calamity, caring for friends and neighbors in trouble, and communicating to ensure solidarity among people important to them.

They were willing to take risks to hold on, reach out to those in need who reciprocated in kind, and become appropriately literate to avoid the perils of ignorance. Each of those characteristics were a way to survive. By staying ahead of problems. By building a cohort of people they could count on. By never doing anything dumb because of ignorance.

Growing up in that setting affected the development of my purpose. I planned, tried to be involved with others, and did what I could to avoid ignorance. But as much as those facets of purpose became important to me, they eventually seemed too inward-looking.

The other three influences found their way into my persona: *culture*, *aptitude*, and *values*.

The *culture* in which I grew up involved exciting post-World War II ideas, events, and products. There was a kind of optimism in the wind, a "can do" attitude of which I wanted to be a part.

My *aptitude*, or potential, became more evident to me. It allowed me to do more with life than just survive. Maybe I could use that potential to serve others.

Values taught by my family were notably impressive, and I appreciated their significance. Religious values played a role in my thinking. But I was curious about value systems emanating from other people and various venues. Out of that milieu came my purpose to be another person's life partner. And a caregiver, no matter what.

Family, culture, aptitude, and values coalesced to be the foundation of my life's purpose. I could not escape it even if I thought I wanted to.

Chapter 37
Culture

Culture has many definitions and must be used in context, especially as we create and pursue our purpose in life. One context pertains to genealogical *family characteristics*:

The culture emanating from family history. Beliefs, interactions of family members, socio-economic levels, customs, techniques for overcoming hardships and meeting opportunity.

A second context is the larger *social environment* within which a family exists:

- neighborhoods, communities, states, nations
- war, peace, poverty, prosperity, disease
- compatibility, prejudice, race, religion
- rural, urban, suburban
- transportation and communication
- technology
- health care and nutrition

The third context involves *time and place*:

As time passes cultures become different. We travel and move to different places. Time and place change our perceptions of cultural influences, sometimes intentionally, often unintentionally.

During the present time it feels as if everything is out of control. Families struggle with unfamiliar issues. The society around us is growing more confrontational and dysfunctional. Time has moved us into an era we do not recognize. The place we once thought we knew is not the same. Our culture is shifting like wet sand on a beach. It is hard to keep our balance.

As a science teacher, my wife marveled at how living things on earth could adjust to changing circumstances. To survive—even thrive by reinventing their cultures. Adjustments in nature rarely occur in a single lifespan. While human beings are no exception, our more powerful brain can refashion responses *within* a lifetime.

We learn. This learning awakens our perspective on what is happening and how we must handle the situation. Nevertheless, we revise our behaviors within the confines of cultural norms deeply ingrained within us.

For example, I became enamored with the military because of its emphasis on discipline, order, and a thrilling esprit de corps purpose. My interest in serving the military did not emanate from a family history that glorified the armed services. But it was compatible with a family and social culture that revered self-discipline and a willingness to sacrifice for a worthwhile cause.

That attitude changed the longer I served in the army and the more I fully comprehended its primary reason for existence. Never disputing the need for a strong military in a dangerous world, I began to think of my service as that of a "citizen soldier." To do what was expected as a patriotic American. To do it well, but nothing more. My culture created in me a need to serve. But how I served affected my ultimate purpose for living.

My wife was raised in a Texas family that revered southern traditions. Food, manners, dress, emphasis on family, church affiliation, Christian belief systems, manners. Many of which seemed like oddities to me, a man raised in Arizona when it still had an Old West feel about it.

In time I grew to appreciate most of the 1962 Texas culture, but not all of it. As a white boy growing up in a state with diverse and often intermixed cultures, I had little experience with segregation, and the army was totally desegregated. At that time of my life, my attitude about segregation in Texas was not based on moral repugnance. It was mostly *I don't get it.*

My wife shared my view. Her parents did not, except for one curious cultural oddity. They were almost obsessively dedicated and loyal to any black or Hispanic person who worked for them in the household or company or were hired to maintain their property. It partially came down to whether minority persons knew and accepted their "place."

My wife held a more-enriched attitude. In the church and community, she often made friends with minority women. Occasionally, the friendship was powerful. When one of those friends died, she insisted that we pay for a beautiful headstone. My wife's openness to people of color made a significant difference in her response to care as an Alzheimer's patient.

Before the pandemic I visited my wife's care facility every day. The bonus received from those visits was watching and listening to other patients and their families. Patients and visitors respond to each other in interesting ways.

The wife of a male resident was once a prominent jurist. She read to him excerpts from the *American Constitution* and *Declaration of Independence*. I could see the vacant look in his eyes momentarily disappear as he listened to his wife recite words that obviously meant much to him. Those words became a cognitive stimulus that represented a culture both admired.

Conversely, one female resident clearly wanted nothing to do with her husband when he visited. Their son told me the marriage had been dysfunctional. The culture of animosity was deeply rooted in her.

Many on the facility's caregiving staff are people of color. Most residents cooperate with them, but the prejudices of a lifetime sometimes emerge through the fog of Alzheimer's. Impatience. The expectation they must be waited on.

The opposite is true with my wife. She smiles and obviously loves and appreciates people taking care of her. Just as she and her parents did for those working for them in that odd, segregated culture. One that had a positive flip side—loving paternalism. Intellectually, my wife understood the dangers of paternalism. She forced herself out of the culture of a superior person taking care of an inferior being.

Recently I mentioned the name "Laura" to my wife, and she smiled contentedly. Laura was a black woman who helped clean our house but was also a wonderful friend. She contracted terminal breast cancer, so my wife and I visited her in the hospital. During our last visit Laura told my wife, "We're like sisters with different mothers."

Funny but true. They had created a new culture for themselves. More than equality. A kinship built on empathy and a deep emotional connection. If only such a cultural bond of mutual understanding and love would develop in all of us during this time of crisis.

Chapter 38
Aptitude

Standardized testing became popular in the twentieth century and is still used today. It categorizes people according to certain traits, particularly their aptitude. The most famous of such tests measures intelligence. Others are used to determine the extent to which someone can perform a job or succeed in a degree program.

Learning all we can is challenging. Mostly trial and error as we grow to adulthood. Tests are designed to overcome our dependence on trial and error. They are meant to efficiently reveal an aptitude we did not realize. A short cut.

Aptitude tests cover two fundamental issues: (1) measuring what they are supposed to measure and (2) consistently measuring potential over time. The first condition is *validity* while the second is *reliability*.

Statisticians can check both validity and reliability within parameters, as in a range of conditions. Like weather forecasters telling us the probability of rain is 30 percent. *Validity* is never 100 percent because written language can be interpreted differently. *Reliability* is never 100% because human moods vary each day.

Other problems surface with aptitude tests. They are weak in assessing a person's abilities across the full spectrum of human personalities and aspirations. Now and in the future. Cultural influences. Past and future emotional experiences. Relationships. Hardships. Mind-altering revelations.

They are not good in predicting the power of ambition, gritty determination to succeed, and acceptance of failure as motivation to do it better next time. Of circumventing traditional approaches to solving problems thereby discovering something entirely new.

Another factor is the self-fulfilling prophecy which can work in both directions. Some do what is prophesied by tests because they are predisposed that way. How can the test be wrong?

For me it worked the opposite way when my sixth-grade teacher said an aptitude test suggested I would be a good accountant. From that point forward I never wanted to be an accountant.

Today, educational psychologists say a test is just one tool to help students discover talents and potential. I agree. When it is a means to stimulate dialogue and reflection, with a full understanding of the test's strengths and deficiencies. But even those conditions may not be enough.

Aptitude is like an internal shapeshifter, looking like one thing today and quite another tomorrow. It becomes a valuable part of who we are only after we are forced to rise to an occasion, to face a challenge and overcome it.

A man against the elements, who almost dies yet succeeds in the face of certain disaster. A woman who finds herself alone after a family tragedy or disruption yet reaches deep into her reservoir of talents to build a new life.

Where do those kinds of aptitude come from? Were they lying below the surface all along, just waiting to be tapped? Why did they not show up earlier?

As educators, my wife and I believed our job was to help students locate the aptitude below the surface and give them confidence to try it out. To use it as much as possible in and outside the classroom. It was more than giving students self-confidence which in immature minds can turn into cognitive or physical bullying.

Finding and using a subsurface aptitude must be channeled into a disciplined and respectful set of behaviors. A quiet yet persistent way of conducting oneself, thereby showing up as thoughtful leadership, caring service, or a creative contribution.

In recent years I have wondered where my aptitude for caregiving comes from. Some would say such an ability is more deeply rooted in innate love than something nurtured from learning experiences. That may be true.

But love is a nebulous emotion that defies precise definition. It involves connectedness and loyalty. The best way I can describe it is in terms of loss. The thing that happens to my innerworkings when I lose someone fully intertwined with my life. Brother. Parents. Other relatives. Friends.

Nevertheless, learning experiences in the context of universal truths and overriding aspects of living must play a role. Maybe it is associated with the acceptance of responsibility.

Can responsibility be an aptitude? Families teach their children to be responsible. As in other forms of educational experiences, some children are quick learners while others are not. Teachers call it readiness.

When are young people ready to define, accept and practice what we know as responsibility? My definition of responsibility is the innate willingness to "be there" when others need help.

In my youth I was much influenced by Isaiah 6:8, *"Then I heard the voice of the Lord saying, 'Whom shall I send? And who will go for us?' And I said, 'Here am I. Send me!'"* (KJV).

Maybe the "be there" idea of accepting responsibility was an aptitude lying just below the surface. Whatever it was and is today, it is something I both accept and absolutely *must* practice. And my wife felt the same way. In many ways, much more so. To "be there" for the deprived, the shunned, the disenfranchised.

In recent months I have seen thousands of others who also have an aptitude for responsibility, at a much greater level than I. This humbles me. It makes me understand how many are being responsible in ways that entail a much greater sacrifice than my own.

It also encourages me, because a few others believe everything bad that happens is someone else's fault. Conversely, everything good that happens is because of their actions.

I long for the time when my wife and I could sit in our den and talk about responsibility as an aptitude. As a couple. As educators who believed schools were being dragged into the training mode of thinking, limited to preparing students for careers in science, technology, engineering, and mathematics. That schools were no longer partners with families in the development of worthwhile values, but preparation academies for business and industry to support a strong economy.

Under the notion that families and churches should be solely responsible for the "soft" values. Defined by some as being inconsequential when compared to making tough decisions. Taking definitive action to preserve the right of individuals to be assertive and presumably effective in a dog-eat-dog world.

Believe me, caregiving is anything but a "soft" value. It requires a kind of toughness that percolates up through the aptitude that lies below the surface of good people.

Chapter 39
Values

Values is another English word with multiple meanings. As a noun it can be defined as wealth, a numerical amount, or moral standards. As a verb it can be an estimate of worth, something or someone to cherish.

What we value typifies who we are and how we behave.

In 1970 my father and I saw the movie, *Patton*. I had served in Patton's armored division sixteen years after his death in 1945. Even in death, Patton's personality pervaded that unit's culture. Patton was born wealthy to a family with a strong military heritage. He was athletic and a historical mystic. As depicted in the movie, Patton saw himself as the modern embodiment of a mythical military past. One in which winning—and ultimate conquering— were the most important goals in life.

After seeing the movie, my father was curious how my military service might have caused me to be more competitive. In my youth I was never competitive. Games were just games. I did not care if I won or lost, did not value winning for the sake of winning.

But to feel successful, winning must matter. Really matter. When lives are at stake. When failure, suffering and pain are the result of losing. I value winning when it means something.

My greatest worry in the army was that I would lose soldiers because of my stupid mistakes. I told myself that conquering a faceless enemy in battle, as much as I accepted that important objective, was less significant than the loss of people who trusted me. Because of an odd set of circumstances, I was never asked to test my values in a shooting war. Main battle tanks were not used by the army in Vietnam.

But as an educator my values have been tested. Overcoming obstacles in the personal as well as the academic growth of students and clients. My values are unfulfilled if I fail to accomplish those goals. And a certain kind of suffering results.

I admire medical professionals. They value healing and feel failure when their skills are not enough. When their patients grow worse and sometimes die. They fear making mistakes that result in pain and suffering— sometimes death.

As the caregiver for my wife who will certainly die from Alzheimer's, I wish my skills as a husband were enough to stop it. But I will lose.

The medical and residential staff will also lose. Our lofty values to *first do no harm*, and then find ways to avoid the inevitable, will be for naught.

An attempt to win over Alzheimer's is like experiences with other terminal diseases and disorders humankind has not conquered. Winning will not happen now, not even in this era.

We do not win over death and some disorders leading to it, no matter how hard we try. Regardless of how often I tell myself that kind of winning is meaningful.

At this stage in our lives, all my wife and I can do is value what we have always valued. Only I can verbalize those values now: Family. Service. Love. My hope is that she is still able to sense those things in her limited consciousness and marginally demonstrated depth of feeling.

The questions I ask myself now are: *What will I value after the caregiving is done? What will I value after my wife dies? How will I act on those values in the remaining years of my life?*

Caregivers die too. Until then, what is the charge, or set of instructions emanating from years of marriage and service to family? Service to other people. Service to the loving connectedness of humankind.

In trying to act on those three goals I start with *family* which is the living, loving result of our marriage. To cement relationships and help build foundations for eternal bonding.

Continuing to *serve others* is more challenging now. As a retired man with no institutional base other than volunteering. So, I volunteer for AARP. Seek ways to further the goals of my church and community. And I write.

The loving connectedness of humankind is possibly the most challenging charge. Probably because I am most acutely aware of love's meaning when

I reflect on loss. Loving connectedness is the overriding meaning of our otherwise finite existence.

⬺⬻

Stephen Hawking and Carl Sagan were scientists, not theologians. They were the world's foremost scholars on matters having to do with the massive universe of which we are just a small part. Both Hawking and Sagan were secularists, in that they neither disputed nor verified the existence of God and a spiritual world.

What fascinated both men, and other scientists like them, is that our bodies are made up of the same stuff that gives the universe shape and substance. In other words, the molecules that exist within us are no different than those of the most remote star or planet. Connectedness.

Toward the end of their lives, both Hawking and Sagan were interviewed extensively on their beliefs about the meaning of our lives and the existence of the universe. *Connectedness* was the point.

Stars and planets are irretrievably connected by the laws of physics. Mostly gravity and motion. Life on earth is connected the same way. Take away just one piece and everything dies. Plants, water, oxygen, climate, and millions of other connections are essential.

The status of our environment has become a vigorous topic of discussion, as it must. It is essential to the survival of the planet on which we exist. But what to do about it is constantly disputed.

The loving connectedness of humankind is also a vital subject. Like the environment, what we should do to ensure its continuance is also disputed.

It boils down to what we value as a means for attaining a goal. Some value the unfettered advancement of human progress as it has evolved in the past. Growth in manufacturing and development. Conquering obstacles. Unfettered entrepreneurship. Solving problems through individual achievement and the competitive spirit.

In many ways I admire those values, and I have exercised them myself. But the kind of connectedness they enshrine are rooted in the chaos theory, which is a mathematical term that accepts the idea a small glitch somewhere can change everything. Glitches have been unacceptable to me as a husband who cares for his wife

A loving connectedness needs to work within a stable universe as much as possible. That is the essence of what I value and will fiercely do anything in my attempt to control it.

That is the uniqueness of our human, loving connectedness. Death will cause us to lose that connectedness we value so much. But until the laws of the universe win, we will stay true to the value of *being there* for each other.

Chapter 40
Compendium

Not many positive spins can be put on Alzheimer's and its effect on both the afflicted and those who care for them. Other publications address the challenges of Alzheimer's with attempts to remain upbeat. They sometimes succeed.

I have attempted to weave an upbeat perspective. One of the best is that *love is a pervasive reality when other forms of cognition have weakened or disappeared.*

No science supports that opinion, but I have seen it happen in my wife and others. It is something sensed intuitively or felt physically. A flicker of a smile. A spoken word that seems to come out of nowhere. A movement of the eyes. The tilt of her head. A strange look of contentment that settles over a body that was once a source of discomfort or great pain.

In my wife I sense something else which makes me especially happy. An aura of *satisfaction* surrounds her. As if the memories of her eighty years are compressed into a kernel of something properly completed. In that tiny space she has stored the richness of many experiences— happy, sad, fulfilling, encouraging, worthwhile.

That expression of satisfaction in my wife helps me believe I played a role. Far from perfect, but enough to nurture her fulfillment. I see much the same thing in others who live in the memory care facility. But not always. It is hard to watch some people who appear to be full of anger, abject disgust, even fear. I do not know their backstories. Maybe they were similar to ours and the brain has just gone topsy-turvy. Credible evidence suggests that possibility.

Who am I to judge? Prior to my wife's current status there were occasions when she demonstrated paranoia, anger, beliefs in false narratives, misjudgments, and other aberrations.

But now, all those issues are gone. And that pleases me.

What about the role of imagination? I like to think my powers of imagination and creativity are okay, maybe even better than average. My imagination is not fantastical but rooted in reality. A little like C.S. Lewis (*The Chronicles of Narnia*) and J. R. R. Tolkien (*The Hobbit* and *The Lord of the Rings*). Both scholars realized their academic publications would reach a larger cohort of readers only if they used figurative expression and metaphor.

When my wife and I read those books or watched the movies, we reacted differently. She was engrossed with the fantasy that allowed her to escape into a different reality. That escape somehow comforted her, decades before her Alzheimer's diagnosis.

The imagery of the stories linked with her spiritual side and feelings of lovely wonderment. For me, the stories were simply interesting fictional analogies for Christian teachings (Lewis) or the horrors of and meditations on the effects of World War I (Tolkien).

Even now, my wife seems to have the ability to integrate a kind of fantastical thought process amid the reality of where she is and why she is there. It does not seem to be spiritual in any specific sense, nor is it linked to religious beliefs or actions. In fact, when she is given communion by our church's pastor there is no response beyond going through the motions. No smile or look of contentment on her face. Nothing is rejected, but it is clear her essence is somewhere else.

It takes me back to the early days of our marriage. Because of military and college requirements, our dating was sporadic and long-distance. Our so-called honeymoon was short and not satisfying to either of us, primarily because she had to return to work, and I was starting graduate school in a few short days.

But in the days and weeks afterward we created albums that included pictures of our travels and family activities during courtship. That album-building activity continued during the first years of our life together and perpetuated into the next decades. She thought it was a magical time and I did too. Her fantasy became mine, and mine became hers. I have heard other young couples report the same experience.

Time erodes those feelings, sometimes greatly. Little by little the magic disappears into ennui or even trauma when illness, addiction, death, poverty, misguided behaviors, and other realities of life appear. As with everyone, that happened to us to some extent. It affected both of us and became magnified when the dementia started to appear.

But now, the magic seems to be coming back to my wife. I do not know how or why, but even in this miserable pandemic I can sense it. Through masks, plexiglass barriers, monitored conversations, and social distancing.

As a caregiving husband the magic is not coming back to me as readily as it did fifty-eight years ago. But the fact I can sense it in her is comforting. I know she is suffering from neither physical nor psychic pain. She exists in a kind of fantasy world in which magic and wonderment completely encompass her. Her smile is almost angelic and her barely audible responses are always words such as "beautiful" and "delightful."

This book and other activities distract me away from a longing to return to the magical life we once had together. Distractions and associations with other people are important and necessary, but nothing is quite enough.

But they will have to suffice for me to be a continuing member of humanity and a productive element of society.

Alzheimer's and
a Guide to the Husband

This last entry is meant to be a guide for you, the men taking care of the women you love. I offer these five suggestions with the knowledge we are different in many ways. You know what those differences are. I have mentioned them often at various points in this book. So please do not think of these "tips" as do's or don'ts. They are meant only for your reflection.

NETWORK. It is all about the team. Everything from a small group of family members to a community of supporters. Get over the idea you are somehow invincible. Trust me, you are not! Recruit, enlist, and search for people beyond the home you share with your wife. Appreciate and welcome children, grandchildren, old friends, neighbors, fellow church or club members, or any responsible person who steps forward and offers assistance.

Many of them will instinctively know what to do. Others will ask you what they can do to help, so make a list of things you are having trouble with. Cooking, cleaning, fixing your wife's hair, bathing her, and helping with other day-to-day tasks. Running errands such as grocery shopping and picking up medications. Giving you a break so you can have coffee with your friends or go bowling.

The team you create will include as many or more women than men, so be sure they know they are appreciated. Nothing big, just expressions of gratitude that quietly come from your heart. That is all they need or want.

MONEY. Get over the embarrassment of not having enough money. Alzheimer's is expensive. It can, like other afflictions that show up out of the blue, quickly wipe out what seems to be a nice retirement nest egg. Do not suffer quietly because you feel like a failure. You are not. But be careful about scammers who will loan you money, then make your financial situation infinitely worse.

Respondents to my blog, *Alzheimer's and the Husband* (www.stuervay. com/blog) have included men not yet retired and therefore qualified for Social Security and Medicare. They care for a wife with early-onset dementia. But even couples who qualify for those governmental support systems are obligated to pay for either in-home or residential assistance out-of-pocket. Both kinds of services can be oppressively expensive.

Find a *reputable* financial advisor through community service organizations, churches, knowledgeable financial institutions, and charitable groups. Include your children and other members of the family in these discussions.

You may be told to use equity available in your home, carefully draw down life insurance policies, and explore methods for accessing investments set aside for retirement. If you had the foresight to purchase long-term care insurance, that can be a big plus. If all those options are insufficient, Medicaid is available as a last resort.

Finally, regardless of your political leanings about the role of government, it only makes sense to stay alert to how the nation and state to which you give allegiance, is giving allegiance back to you. This is especially true of veterans and others, such as first responders who have served while in harm's way.

FITNESS. Some men literally kill themselves caring for their wives. A few will die before their wives do. Often a man's decline is because he has underlying conditions or debilitating illnesses of his own.

Sometimes an otherwise healthy guy is stubborn enough to ignore his stress. Or he turns to alcohol or some other addictive substance to get him through each day. Eating habits go haywire, and the lounge chair in front of the TV looks good after the wife is finally asleep. But lounge chair sleep is not relaxing. It is a stupor acquired from psychic and physical exhaustion. Day after day.

It is easy to think that remaining personally fit is not high on the list of remedies for grief and depression. That is a big mistake. But involvement with fitness is sometimes difficult. Walking around the block may be out of the question, because leaving the wife alone is risky. Exercise machines can help if there is household space and discipline enough to use them. Personal trainers are available to guide an exercise regimen virtually, but they are expensive.

My answer has been using stretch exercises and being careful about my diet. The rationale involves not only my health, but adequacy in taking care of my wife's needs. Writing keeps my mind active, but those with other important skills should remain involved with them. Some might refer to them as distractions, but they let the brain go somewhere else for a task-oriented respite.

My most recent distraction was the decision to give up maintenance-free living and buy a home with my sons in a location that supports family gatherings. I can do a little work in the house and yard, enough to keep me focused on the more mundane aspects of living. To the young and healthy, "mundane" is boring. But for caregivers, it can be a lifesaver.

LOVE. Throughout this book I have made frequent references to love. It has been referred to as a nebulous and indefinable thing, like the air we breathe. Like air, love is essential to human life.

But it can be complex and hard to manage. Some manipulate in the name of love. Others demonstrate so much emotion that expressions of love become debilitating, and timid acquiescence only elicits disdain. Those behaviors are not my definition of love.

If nurtured over time, real love has a *regenerative* quality that makes it possible to perpetuate the romantic love we once had for our young, beautiful, and quick-witted brides. Into the years she slowly becomes physically and mentally different. Into the last few years in which she fades away with Alzheimer's.

Regenerative love has many parts but is fundamentally based on a sensitive awareness of life's vicissitudes. What transforms us physically and mentally is not reflective of our inner core. The interior spirit or life force that makes us who we really are.

My wife remains, even in the grip of Alzheimer's, the same caring and purposeful person she has always been. Her essence is regenerated even now, and so must my love for her.

BELONG. Belonging to something bigger than you are.

At one time belonging was easier than it is now. While growing up, most adults belonged to churches, clubs, service organizations, and social groups. They were more than just enjoyable diversions. Those activities gave people an opportunity to expand their social horizons and absorb benefits that come from a sense of place. They also benefitted the community in general.

Social and entertainment media have in many ways replaced those outlets, especially during a pandemic. My involvement with AARP and church is as much a way to serve my own emotional needs as it is a way to serve others. They are mutually dependent.

I must continue to belong, because to let myself become isolated is one step closer to my own decline That is unacceptable — especially as the caregiver for a wife with Alzheimer's who needs my support.

Epilogue

THE LIFE OF BARBARA PRAEGER ERVAY:
THE JOY OF MAKING A REAL DIFFERENCE!

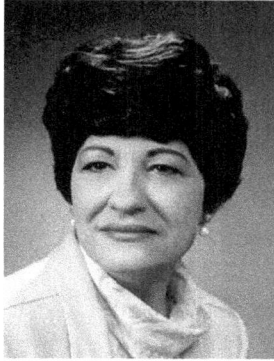

August 10, 1940 – February 5, 2021

According to David Brooks, *New York Times* columnist and author, there is a difference between living a happy life and one filled with joy.

God gives us many ways to be happy if we are willing to open ourselves to the wonders around us. Barbara took advantage of those opportunities.

Barbara Praeger Ervay was indeed happy because she was willing to actively be involved in life. She was born into a loving and supportive family, which she never took for granted. Her parents, Charles and Mary V. Praeger, gave her a comfortable home and as many opportunities as possible to become nurtured and well-educated. Her brother, Chuck, was an important part of Barbara's life. She enjoyed wonderful relationships with many others in her large extended Texas family, including a cousin who was more like a sister, Jayne Chamberlin.

After graduating from Austin College, Barbara married Stuart (Stu) Ervay, an army officer stationed at Fort Hood, Texas. She began her teaching career in Arlington, Texas, then moved with her husband to Irving. Later the family relocated to Scottsdale, Arizona; Denton, Texas; and Emporia, Kansas, where Stu became a professor at Emporia State University. Along the way Barbara brought two outstanding sons into the world: David Blaine Ervay and Corey Edward Ervay.

After relocating to Emporia, Barbara told Stu, "All my goals to achieve happiness have been attained. I'm not sure what else is expected of me, other than raising our children in a happy and cheerful home."

Barbara began the transition from a happy life to one that entailed a sense of joy in herself and those around her. Something much larger than herself—to make a real difference.

Barbara started her quest for joyful fulfillment through church, university and community affiliations. In a few years she had moved into leadership roles as President of the City Women's Club of Emporia, Faculty Wives Club at ESU, Presbyterian Church Women at the church, and the local Beta Sigma Phi chapter. She also became a den mother for the local Cub Scout Pack and organized neighborhood children as helpers with her new passion: gardening and canning food.

Family vacations and holiday gatherings were highlights. Trips to Texas, Arizona, and Ohio. In the summer of 1976, the family celebrated America's Bicentennial by spending three weeks exploring the eastern coast of the U.S. With Barbara's minor field of studies in history, she was a strong contributor to the daily narrative. Spurred on by Barbara, the family became involved in the Boy Scout program. Both David and Corey achieved the rank of Eagle Scout.

Barbara enrolled the family in a foreign exchange program for high school students. Peter Stadelund was a high school student from Denmark, and he joined the family for a year to attend Emporia High

School. Peter also traveled with the family in various parts of the nation. He taught himself, and all the Ervays, about the importance of an international perspective.

After both sons completed high school Barbara had more time to make other connections. She served as a substitute teacher in Emporia and later as a full-time teacher in the North Lyon County Schools. Her contributions as a teacher in Americus Elementary School brought out her special skills, which included supporting students emotionally through the turbulent middle school years. The girls especially needed strong support in a culture that valued male participation in sports, hunting, and other outdoor pursuits. The full extent of Barbara's contribution was realized many years later.

At Barbara's favorite hair salon, a new receptionist recognized the name, Mrs. Ervay. She had been one of Barbara's students in Americus. She told Stu and Barbara about a Facebook group of past Americus students who called themselves, "The Mrs. Ervay Fan Club."

All of those women, now in their 40s, had been greatly influenced by Barbara. They believed she made them more confident, positive, and happy. She believed in them and was supportive even after they moved on to high school and beyond.

In the latter half of the 1980s Barbara decided to end public-school teaching. She began master's degree studies in school leadership, curriculum, and instruction. She also worked two years as a graduate assistant in ESU's Department of School Leadership. After receiving her master's degree in school leadership, Barbara continued work toward an educational specialist degree, a program that was discontinued before she could complete the requirements. Nevertheless, that activity placed her in a position to work with regular faculty members as they pursued various research interests.

Research topics prominent at the time were those associated with supporting women interested in educational leadership. Barbara worked with faculty members and fellow students, conducting research and writing articles. She became more interested in how the Presbyterian Church supported women and people from diverse cultural backgrounds.

Stu noticed that the Presbytery of Northern Kansas was forming a Committee on Women's Concerns, with a similar group formed at the Synod (state) level. Barbara immediately joined those committees and soon found herself in leadership roles. Later she attended the Triennial Churchwide Gathering of Presbyterian Women. She studied the issues carefully, led many workshops, and wrote articles. She felt as if she was making a real difference. There is no doubt she did because the role of women in the church is much different today than it was thirty years ago.

In the meantime, other needs became part of Barbara's life. She helped her parents in San Antonio manage problems associated with their aging. Her mother was beginning to show signs of dementia and her father was becoming blind. It was impossible to move to Texas, but Barbara spent plenty of time on the road. She arranged for and oversaw caregiving activities. It was physically and emotionally stressful, but she got the job done.

In the early 1990s, Stu formed an organization called the Curriculum Leadership Institute. Barbara was a sounding board as the idea was conceptualized, and she worked hard to assist. Her graduate studies were invaluable to Stu and others as they slowly created the service and publishing organization that has since helped hundreds of school districts around the nation.

The joy of making a real difference is Barbara's legacy. Her legacy is further enhanced by the love and dedication shown to her family, and her enormous interest in learning more about her faith and the world around us. She was a Christian, Presbyterian, wife, mother, teacher of science and history, researcher, and student and practitioner of altruism in its best applications.

Stu often said, "The best of many characteristics I saw in Barbara after dating her two or three times was how much she cared for those who were rejected or sidelined by others."

Barbara cared. And all of us loved her for who she was and the contributions she made to our lives and the lives of others. She will be missed.

Acknowledgements

The primary reason this book was written is to honor the life of Barbara Praeger Ervay, my wife of fifty-eight years. Her life was shared with mine, leaving me with the many insights I try to reveal in this manuscript. Together we brought into the world my two best friends — our sons who with their families have supported us in more ways than I can count: David and Debra Ervay, Corey and Gina Ervay. And the grandchildren they gave us: Steven, Kaylin and Megan.

Inspiration has also come from our parents, Francis and Dorothy Ervay and Charles and Mary V. Praeger. I still feel the loving presence of my brother Steve who died in 1973. And I appreciate the love and support from his widow, Judie, and their daughters Amy and Stacey.

Barbara's brother Chuck died during the writing of this book, but he and his wife Denece, with their daughters Leslie and Laura, played a significant part in who and what we were and are as a family.

I am also grateful for the many friends we gained during our life together. While too many to name here, they know who they are and how much they are loved.

Finally, this book would have never been written if it had not been for the patient and understanding help of my editor, RJ Thesman.

About the Author

Stu Ervay is a retired university professor and consultant to public schools. Prior to his work in higher education, he served as a unit commander in the United States Army, and taught history and government in secondary schools.

During his forty-three years of university service, Stu wrote professional books including *The Curriculum Leader* and *Common Sense About the Common Core*. His articles have been published by many educational journals, including The *Oxford Round Table Review*, *NASSP Bulletin*, *Malaysian Journal of Education*, *The Rural Educator*, *Educational Considerations*, *The Teacher Educator*, *Occasional Report*, *American Middle School Education*, *Journal of the Kansas Council for the Social Studies*, *Focus*, *Kansas School Board Journal*, *The Teacher Educator*, *The Educational Forum*, *Phi Delta Kappan*, *Action In Teacher Education*, *Educational Leadership*, *Clearing House*, *Kansas Teacher*, and *Arizona Teacher*.

Stu was founder and first editor of The *Kansas Teacher Education Advocate* and conducted hundreds of workshops and presentations at multiple professional conferences. He was also an Executive Board member in the Association of Teacher Educators. Stu was director of the Emporia State University Office for Professional Education Services, chaired the ESU Department of School Leadership, and was executive director of the ESU Center for Educational Research and Service. He also served as assistant dean of The Teachers College.

While at ESU, Stu led research and development activities that resulted in the 1991 development of a nationally recognized school improvement service, the Curriculum Leadership Institute www.cliweb.org. CLI is a nonprofit publication and service organization that has served hundreds of school districts throughout the nation. CLI leaders are now developing systems to help teachers become more effective as virtual instructors.

Since retirement Stu has written journal articles and a book on school improvement, *The Teacher as Somebody: Skills that Make Teaching a True Profession*. He is now a state AARP volunteer leader and recipient of the *2020 Ann Garvin Award for Excellence in Community Service*. He is also leading an effort to create an AARP Lifespan Planning Course for use in post-secondary institutions and higher education.

His wife, Barbara, is also a retired educator. In addition to many years of teaching middle school science, she played a significant role as an advocate for women in church leadership. Barbara also worked closely with Stu in the development of the Curriculum Leadership Institute

The couple has two sons and three grandchildren. Barbara was diagnosed with Alzheimer's Syndrome in 2014 and is now a resident of a memory care home.

Endnotes

[1] Shaw, George Bernard, *Back to Methuselah*, act I, *Selected Plays with Prefaces*, vol. 2, p. 7 (1949).

[2] Yelln, Keith, *Battle Exhortation: The Rhetoric of Combat Leadership*, (Columbia, S.C.: University of South Carolina Press, Reprint Edition 2011), 64.

[3] AARP and National Alliance for Caregiving. *Caregiving in the United States 2020*. Washington, DC: AARP. May 2020. www.doi.org/10.26419/ppi.00103.001

Picture Credits

Front cover: iStockphoto/monkeybusinessimages

Back cover: iStockphoto/a_Taiga

Picture 1 (Mandy Shoemaker/Michala Gibson) Prairie Elder Care, Overland Park KS 2015.
Company Photo: 10034 West 151st Street, Overland Park, Kansas 66221

Picture 2 (Stu Ervay/Barbara Praeger) Fort Hood, Texas. May 1962.
Photographer: 2nd Lieutenant Don Michael Ogg, 1938-2008.

Picture 3 (Stu, Barbara, David, Corey Ervay) San Antonio, Texas, June 1974.
Photographer: Charles E. Praeger, Jr. 1911-1998

Picture 4 (Barbara and Stu Ervay) Emporia, Kansas, May 1987
Photographer: Corey Ervay

Picture 5 (Ervay Family at Stu's Retirement) Emporia, Kansas, May 2014
Photographer: Stacie Mendenhall

Picture 6 (Barbara) Prairie Elder Care, Overland Park, Kansas, December 2019
Photographer: Stu Ervay

Picture 7 (Barbara) Prairie Elder Care, Overland Park, Kansas, January 2019
Photographer: Stu Ervay

Picture 8 (Barbara, Stu, David, Corey) Prairie Elder Care, Overland Park, Kansas, September 2018. Photographer: Steven Ervay

Picture 9 (Barbara and Stu) Prairie Elder Care, Overland Park, Kansas, August 2019
Photographer: Mandy Shoemaker

Picture 10 (Barbara) Prairie Elder Care, Overland Park, Kansas, August 2020
Photographer: Mandy Shoemaker

Picture 11 (Barbara) Prairie Elder Care, Overland Park, Kansas, February 2020
Photographer: Mandy Shoemaker

www.ingramcontent.com/pod-product-compliance
Lightning Source LLC
Chambersburg PA
CBHW070110030426
42335CB00016B/2093